Medical and Surgical Management of the Diabetic Foot and Ankle

Editor

PETER A. BLUME

CLINICS IN PODIATRIC MEDICINE AND SURGERY

www.podiatric.theclinics.com

Consulting Editor
THOMAS ZGONIS

January 2014 • Volume 31 • Number 1

ELSEVIER

1600 John F. Kennedy Boulevard • Suite 1800 • Philadelphia, Pennsylvania, 19103-2899

http://www.theclinics.com

CLINICS IN PODIATRIC MEDICINE AND SURGERY Volume 31, Number 1
January 2014 ISSN 0891-8422, ISBN-13: 978-0-323-26408-2

Editor: Jennifer Flynn-Briggs

Clinics in Podiatric Medicine and Surgery (ISSN 0891-8422) is published quarterly by Elsevier Inc., 360 Park Avenue South, New York, NY 10010-1710. Months of issue are January, April, July, and October. Business and Editorial Offices: 1600 John F. Kennedy Blvd., Ste. 1800, Philadelphia, PA 19103-2899. Customer Service Office: 3251 Riverport Lane, Maryland Heights, MO 63043. Periodicals postage paid at New York, NY and additional mailing offices. Subscription prices are $305.00 per year for US individuals, $450.00 per year for US institutions, $155.00 per year for US students and residents, $370.00 per year for Canadian individuals, $544.00 for Canadian institutions, $435.00 for international individuals, $544.00 per year for international institutions and $220.00 per year for Canadian and foreign students/residents. To receive student/resident rate, orders must be accompanied by name of affiliated institution, date of term, and the *signature* of program/residency coordinator on institution letterhead. Orders will be billed at individual rate until proof of status is received. Foreign air speed delivery is included in all *Clinics* subscription prices. All prices are subject to change without notice. POSTMASTER: Send address changes to *Clinics in Podiatric Medicine and Surgery*, Elsevier Health Sciences Division, Subscription Customer Service, 3251 Riverport Lane, Maryland Heights, MO 63043. **Customer Service: 1-800-654-2452 (US). From outside of the US, call 314-447-8871. Fax: 314-447-8029. E-mail: JournalsCustomerService-usa@elsevier.com (for print support); JournalsOnlineSupport-usa@elsevier.com (for online support).**

Reprints. For copies of 100 or more of articles in this publication, please contact the Commercial Reprints Department, Elsevier Inc., 360 Park Avenue South, New York, NY 10010-1710. Tel.: 212-633-3874; Fax: 212-633-3820; E-mail: reprints@elsevier.com.

Clinics in Podiatric Medicine and Surgery is covered in *MEDLINE/PubMed (Index Medicus)* and *EMBASE/Excerpta Medica*.

Printed and bound by CPI Group (UK) Ltd, Croydon, CR0 4YY

Transferred to digital print 2012

CLINICS IN PODIATRIC MEDICINE AND SURGERY

CONSULTING EDITOR
THOMAS ZGONIS, DPM, FACFAS

Contributors

CONSULTING EDITOR

THOMAS ZGONIS, DPM, FACFAS
Associate Professor, Division of Podiatric Medicine and Surgery, Department of Orthopaedic Surgery, University of Texas Health Science Center at San Antonio, San Antonio, Texas

EDITOR

PETER A. BLUME, DPM, FACFAS
Assistant Clinical Professor of Surgery, Orthopedics and Rehabilitation, and Anesthesia, Yale School of Medicine, New Haven, Connecticut

AUTHORS

HOMAN BADRI, DPM
Clinical Fellow in Surgery, Mount Auburn Hospital, Harvard Medical School, Cambridge, Massachusetts

TZVI BAR-DAVID, DPM, FACFAS
Division of Podiatric Surgery, Department of Orthopaedic Surgery, Columbia University Medical Center, New York, New York

PETER A. BLUME, DPM, FACFAS
Assistant Clinical Professor of Surgery, Orthopedics and Rehabilitation, and Anesthesia, Yale School of Medicine, New Haven, Connecticut

TROY J. BOFFELI, DPM, FACFAS
Director, Foot and Ankle Surgical Residency Program, Regions Hospital/HealthPartners Institute for Education and Research, Minnesota

JASON A. CHIN, MD
Section of Vascular Surgery, Yale University School of Medicine, New Haven, Connecticut

GAUTHAM CHITRAGARI, MBBS
Section of Vascular Surgery, Department of Surgery, Yale University School of Medicine, New Haven, Connecticut

EMILY A. COOK, DPM, MPH
Clinical Instructor in Surgery, Mount Auburn Hospital, Harvard Medical School, Cambridge, Massachusetts

JEREMY J. COOK, DPM, MPH
Clinical Instructor in Surgery, Mount Auburn Hospital, Harvard Medical School, Cambridge, Massachusetts

RYAN DONEGAN, DPM, MS
Second Year Resident, Section of Podiatric Surgery, Department of Orthopedics and Rehabilitation, Yale New Haven Hospital, New Haven, Connecticut

ROBERT FRIDMAN, DPM, FACFAS
Division of Podiatric Surgery, Department of Orthopaedic Surgery, Columbia University Medical Center, New York, New York

STEWART KAMEN, DPM, FACFAS
Division of Podiatric Surgery, Department of Orthopaedic Surgery, Columbia University Medical Center, New York, New York

DAVID K. LEUNG, MD, PhD
Department of Radiology, Columbia University Medical Center, New York, New York

DAVID B. MAHLER, CPO
Section of Podiatry, Department of Orthopedic Surgery, Yale University School of Medicine, New Haven, Connecticut

SABINA MALHOTRA, DPM
San Diego, California

BRANT L. MCCARTAN, DPM, MBA, MS
Chief Resident, Division of Podiatry, Beth Israel Deaconess Medical Center, Harvard Medical School, Boston, Massachusetts; Private Practice, Milwaukee Foot Specialists, New Berlin, Wisconsin

JOHN MOSTAFA, DPM
Clinical Fellow in Surgery, Mount Auburn Hospital, Harvard Medical School, Cambridge, Massachusetts

MICHAEL J. RASIEJ, MD
Department of Radiology, Columbia University Medical Center, New York, New York

BARRY I. ROSENBLUM, DPM, FACFAS
Assistant Clinical Professor, Surgery, Harvard Medical School, Beth Israel Deaconess Medical Center, Harvard Medical Center, Boston, Massachusetts

BRYAN A. SAGRAY, DPM
Permanente Medical Group, Department of Orthopaedics, Modesto/Stockton, California

BRIAN M. SCHMIDT, DPM
Second Year Resident, Section of Podiatric Surgery, Department of Orthopedics and Rehabilitation, Yale New Haven Hospital, New Haven, Connecticut

STEPHEN M. SCHROEDER, DPM, FACFAS
Sports Medicine Oregon, Tigard, Oregon

SHERIF Y. SHALABY, MD
Postdoctoral Fellow, Department of Vascular Surgery, Yale University School of Medicine, New Haven, Connecticut

RONALD B. STARON, MD, FACR
Department of Radiology, Columbia University Medical Center, New York, New York

JOHN S. STEINBERG, DPM, FACFAS
Associate Professor, Department of Plastic Surgery, Georgetown University School of Medicine; Program Director, MedStar Washington Hospital Center; Podiatric Residency Co-Director, Center for Wound Healing, MedStar Georgetown University Hospital, Washington DC

BAUER E. SUMPIO, MD, PhD, FACS
Professor of Surgery and Radiology, Chief, Section of Vascular Surgery, Department of Surgery, Yale University School of Medicine, New Haven, Connecticut

BRANDON J. SUMPIO, BS
Department of Surgery, Yale University School of Medicine, New Haven, Connecticut

JONATHAN C. THOMPSON, DPM, MHA
Chief Resident, Foot and Ankle Surgical Residency Program, Regions Hospital/HealthPartners Institute for Education and Research, Minnesota

Contents

Foreword: Medical and Surgical Management of the Diabetic Foot and Ankle   xiii

Thomas Zgonis

Preface: Medical and Surgical Management of the Diabetic Foot and Ankle   xv

Peter A. Blume

**Perioperative Management of the Patient with Diabetes Mellitus: Update
and Overview**   1

Stephen M. Schroeder

Perioperative management of diabetic patients involves optimizing glycemic control and negotiating comorbidities to help reduce complications and obtain results on par with nondiabetics. These goals are usually achievable in the elective surgical setting, but they can be more difficult to control in urgent or emergent situations. Understanding and recognizing the comorbidities associated with diabetes is imperative for optimizing outcomes. Regulating hyperglycemia can reduce morbidity, mortality, and postoperative infections. Understanding the effects of cardiac and renal disease is also important. Taking a team approach in managing these complex patients leads to improved outcomes and is now considered the standard of care.

Diabetes Mellitus and Peripheral Vascular Disease: Diagnosis and Management   11

Jason A. Chin and Bauer E. Sumpio

Diabetes mellitus and peripheral artery disease are prevalent diseases throughout the world and often present simultaneously in the same patient, which has direct implications for their diagnosis and management. Refinements of existing and development of new diagnostic and treatment modalities are changing the management of these diseases. This article reviews the significant pathologic basis, history, and physical examination findings with respect to each disease and their presentation together. Advantages and disadvantages of different diagnostic modalities, including noninvasive studies and imaging technologies, are discussed. General medical management principles and indications, techniques, and efficacy of surgical and endovascular interventions are reviewed.

New Modalities in the Chronic Ischemic Diabetic Foot Management   27

Sherif Y. Shalaby, Peter A. Blume, and Bauer E. Sumpio

The diabetic population is increasing worldwide at a staggering rate. Diabetic foot ulcers are a major contributor to nontraumatic lower limb amputations and peripheral arterial disease is one of main contributing pathophysiologic causes of diabetic ulcers. The dire need to reduce complication and wound healing recovery period of the chronic ischemic diabetic foot (CIDF) is indispensable to limb salvage and improvement of quality of life of patients with CIDF. This article discusses newer modalities that have been proposed to improve CIDF efficiently, safely, and effectively either alone or as adjuvants to conventional therapy.

Imaging of Diabetic Foot Infections   43

Robert Fridman, Tzvi Bar-David, Stewart Kamen, Ronald B. Staron,
David K. Leung, and Michael J. Rasiej

> Complications from diabetic foot infections are a leading cause of nontraumatic lower-extremity amputations. Nearly 85% of these amputations result from an infected foot ulcer. Osteomyelitis is present in approximately 20% of diabetic foot infections. It is imperative that clinicians make quick and successful diagnoses of diabetic foot osteomyelitis (DFO) because a delay in treatment may lead to worsening outcomes. Imaging studies, such as plain films, bone scans, musculoskeletal ultrasound, computerized tomography scans, magnetic resonance imaging, and positron emission tomography scans, aid in the diagnosis. However, there are several mimickers of DFO, which present problems to making a correct diagnosis.

Current Therapies for Diabetic Foot Infections and Osteomyelitis   57

Bryan A. Sagray, Sabina Malhotra, and John S. Steinberg

> Treatment of the patient with a diabetic foot infection and underlying osteomyelitis is currently an evolving process, often complicated by neuropathy, peripheral vascular disease, and renal insufficiency. Understanding which patients require hospitalization, intravenous antibiotic therapy, and urgent operative intervention may ultimately prevent the spread of infection or major limb amputation. The treating surgeon should focus on accurate and early diagnosis, proper antibiosis, and appropriate surgical debridement to eradicate infection while preserving function with a plantar-grade foot.

Offloading of the Diabetic Foot: Orthotic and Pedorthic Strategies   71

Brant L. McCartan and Barry I. Rosenblum

> The diabetic foot is more susceptible than the non-diabetic foot to collapse. This frequently leads to bony prominences followed by ulceration. Offloading of areas of increased pressure is paramount to ulcer prevention and healing. Several devices and accommodations can aid practitioners in saving patients' extremities and allow them to ambulate. A team approach works best, and patient education is a must. Regular assessment and modifications are required for longevity of each device. In this article, different therapeutic options are detailed. A variety of presentations and situations are discussed and the authors' best tips for avoiding complications are offered.

Bioengineered Alternative Tissues   89

Emily A. Cook, Jeremy J. Cook, Homan Badri, and John Mostafa

> Bioengineered alternative tissues (BATs) are heterogeneous processed materials used to aid in wound closure of diabetic foot ulcers. There has been significant progress in the development and clinical use of BATs in the last decade. BATs may be derived from an autograft, allograft, or xenograft source. They may be a single-layer material and consist of only an epidermal or dermal component or they may be bilayer, consisting of both epidermal and dermal components. The holy grail of tissue replacement has yet to be discovered. Nevertheless, if researchers and

bioengineers can flip the switch to return cells to their prenatal period, this can be a breakthrough in cellular regeneration.

Partial Foot Amputations for Salvage of the Diabetic Lower Extremity 103

Troy J. Boffeli and Jonathan C. Thompson

Lower extremity infections are a common yet unfortunate complication of diabetes-related ulcers often requiring surgical intervention. The main goals of surgical treatment consist of selecting the appropriate procedure to effectively eradicate nonsalvageable tissue, achieve primary healing, and maximize subsequent dynamic functionality. An overview of each partial foot amputation procedure is discussed with a focus on procedure selection as well as standard and advanced surgical techniques. The effective application of partial foot amputations in the high-risk diabetic population can act to minimize the need for major proximal lower limb amputations.

The Role of Plastic Surgery for Soft Tissue Coverage of the Diabetic Foot and Ankle 127

Peter A. Blume, Brian M. Schmidt, and Ryan Donegan

The goal of wound healing is to obtain the best closure through the least morbid means. In the surgical treatment of the diabetic foot and ankle, the reconstructive foot and ankle surgeon is tasked with the challenge of repairing a variety of tissue defects. The decision for wound closure depends on the location of the wound and host factors. In order of increasing complexity, the clinician should consider the reconstruction decision ladder algorithm. Wound evaluation coupled with the knowledge of various closure techniques and their indications will arm the surgeon with the tools for a successful closure.

Charcot Neuroarthropathy of the Foot and Ankle: Diagnosis and Management Strategies 151

Peter A. Blume, Bauer Sumpio, Brian Schmidt, and Ryan Donegan

This article reviews current literature discussing the etiology, pathophysiology, diagnosis and imaging, and conservative and surgical treatment of Charcot osteoarthropathy. The treatment of Charcot osteoarthropathy with concurrent osteomyelitis is also discussed.

Prosthetic Options Available for the Diabetic Lower Limb Amputee 173

Gautham Chitragari, David B. Mahler, Brandon J. Sumpio, Peter A. Blume, and Bauer E. Sumpio

Although the rate of lower limb amputation in patients with diabetes is decreasing, amputation still remains a major complication of diabetes. Prosthetics have been long used to help amputees ambulate. The last decade has seen many advances in prostheses with the enhanced understanding of the mechanics of ambulation and improved use of technology. This review describes the different types of prosthetic options available for below knee, ankle, and foot amputees, emphasizing the latest advances in prosthetic design.

Index 187

CLINICS IN PODIATRIC MEDICINE AND SURGERY

FORTHCOMING ISSUES

April 2014
Hallux Abducto Valgus Surgery
Babek Baravarian, *Editor*

July 2014
Adult Acquired Flatfoot Deformity
Alan R. Catanzariti, DPM and
Robert W. Mendicino, DPM, *Editors*

October 2014
**Lower Extremity Complex
Trauma and Complications**
John J. Stapleton, *Editor*

RECENT ISSUES

October 2013
Pediatric Foot Deformities
Patrick DeHeer, *Editor*

July 2013
Advances in Forefoot Surgery
Charles M. Zelen, DPM, *Editor*

April 2013
Revision Total Ankle Replacement
Thomas S. Roukis, DPM, *Editor*

January 2013
Primary Total Ankle Replacement
Thomas S. Roukis, DPM, *Editor*

DOWNLOAD Free App!

Review Articles
THE CLINICS

NOW AVAILABLE FOR YOUR iPhone and iPad

Foreword

Medical and Surgical Management of the Diabetic Foot and Ankle

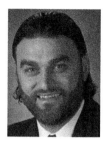

Thomas Zgonis, DPM, FACFAS
Consulting Editor

This edition of *Clinics in Podiatric Medicine and Surgery* is focused on the medical and surgical management of the diabetic foot and ankle. The incidence of diabetic foot pathology and its related devastating complications from neuropathic foot ulceration to Charcot neuroarthropathy has exponentially increased in the United States and around the world. A variety of complications including critical limb ischemia, diabetic foot infections, osteomyelitis, Charcot neuroarthropathy, and amputations are well covered by the experienced invited authors and guest editor Dr Peter Blume. Additional topics include plastic reconstruction and off-loading techniques for the diabetic foot as well as the use of bioengineered alternative tissues for soft tissue coverage of the diabetic foot.

The importance of a multidisciplinary team model in any academic or private practice is also well emphasized throughout this issue. This concept has been well proven in many scientific studies for the overall medical and surgical management of the patient with diabetes mellitus. Patient care education and prevention are also key points to the patient's successful treatment by understanding the devastating multiple organ

Clin Podiatr Med Surg 31 (2014) xiii–xiv
http://dx.doi.org/10.1016/j.cpm.2013.11.001
0891-8422/14/$ – see front matter © 2014 Published by Elsevier Inc.

podiatric.theclinics.com

failures of diabetes mellitus. Finally, I would like to thank the invited authors and guest editor for their outstanding contributions.

Thomas Zgonis, DPM, FACFAS
Division of Podiatric Medicine and Surgery
Department of Orthopaedic Surgery
University of Texas Health Science Center San Antonio
7703 Floyd Curl Drive, MSC 7776
San Antonio, TX 78229, USA

E-mail address:
zgonis@uthscsa.edu

Preface

Medical and Surgical Management of the Diabetic Foot and Ankle

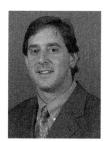

Peter A. Blume, DPM, FACFAS
Editor

The medical and surgical management of the diabetic foot and ankle is a broad topic that involves the crucial multidisciplinary medical team. The evolution of the multidisciplinary approach toward limb preservation requires the knowledge and skill sets of numerous medical professionals. The medical management of the diabetic foot and ankle is paramount to a successful surgical outcome for each and every member of the team.

In this issue of *Clinics in Podiatric Medicine and Surgery*, the broad range of topics will enable all readers to comprehend the importance of medical and surgical management strategies for salvage of the diabetic foot and ankle. The perioperative management of patients with diabetes mellitus is a topic that involves many end-organ diseases with multiple comorbidities. The strategies for management of patients with diabetes during the perioperative period can provide much improved outcomes for salvage options.

Limb preservation would not be possible without vascular intervention. The ability to diagnose and manage peripheral arterial disease has significantly improved over the past several years. The noninvasive testing mechanisms, strategies for identifying disease patterns of arterial disease in the lower extremities, and the advancement of endovascular reconstruction have provided patients with improved circulation and thus require additional wound care and tissue coverage for these complex individuals. Distal revascularization can be achieved with an open standard approach in addition to percutaneous procedures.

The ability to image the diabetic foot and ankle is presented as an updated review with respect to the new modalities and outcomes for sensitivities and specificities. The identification of underlying osteomyelitis, osteoarthropathy, and soft tissue and bone pathology will allow practitioners the ability to proceed with planned strategies.

The current thought process for diabetic foot infections and osteomyelitis has evolved with newer antibiotic therapies, debridement techniques, and a renewed

Clin Podiatr Med Surg 31 (2014) xv–xvi
http://dx.doi.org/10.1016/j.cpm.2013.10.001
0891-8422/14/$ – see front matter © 2014 Elsevier Inc. All rights reserved.

podiatric.theclinics.com

experience with cherished procedures. Resistant-bacterial pathogens are treated with numerous agents that have recently become available and provide options for eradication of these returning bacterial species.

The treatment algorithm for diabetic foot and ankle wounds with respect to bioengineered alternative tissues has become ever so important with limb-preservation techniques. These tissues are an important adjunct therapy for many wounds associated with the diabetic foot and ankle. They have provided coverage options for these very challenging wounds and thus enhance the limb preservation outcome.

Partial foot amputations continue to play an important role in salvage of the diabetic lower extremity. The underlying biomechanics of each amputation are well-known in the podiatric foot and ankle arena. Each of these partial foot amputations provides an option for continued limb salvage. The partial foot amputation can provide a long-term and sustainable outcome for bipedal motion. This topic has enormous importance as many limbs can successfully undergo revascularization even in the high-risk populations due to endovascular reconstruction.

The role of plastic surgery for soft tissue coverage of the diabetic foot and ankle is a field of its own. I originally wrote and was the guest editor for Plastic Surgery: Part 1 and Plastic Surgery: Part 2 in April and October 2000. We now understand the importance of plastic surgery for limb preservation. The reconstructive options have expanded with the broader indications for flap and skin grafting of the diabetic foot and ankle. Negative pressure therapy and tissue biologics in addition to improved angiosome targeting for revascularization have created a broader wound bed for final plastic and reconstructive surgery. The adaptation of many fasciocutaneous flaps for foot and ankle reconstruction are now well-known in the community of limb preservation. Local flaps and split-thickness skin grafts can provide broad coverage options for tissue deficits and chronic wounds of the diabetic foot and ankle.

The diagnosis and management of Charcot neuroarthropathy has also transitioned over the past several years. External fixation, flap management, newer fixation techniques both internal and external, offloading, and a variety of adjunct treatments have allowed practitioners to salvage and preserve more limbs that are plagued with neuroarthropathy. This complicated disease process associated with diabetes mellitus and peripheral neuropathy can be devastating for this group of individuals. This article updates practitioners on a variety of options available for treatment of Charcot neuroarthropathy.

The practitioners who provide care within the limb preservation community must understand the importance of prosthetic management for the diabetic amputee. Many of these problems associated with diabetic foot and ankle disease require some form of prosthetic offloading. Bracing, shoe gear modification, orthotic fabrication, partial or complete foot amputation, or below- and above-knee amputation require the knowledge and availability of an individual with a skill set commensurate with each level of disability.

This updated journey for medical and surgical management of the diabetic foot and ankle provides practitioners with a comprehensive overview of this extremely important topic. I would hope that each practitioner who reads this *Clinics in Podiatric Medicine and Surgery* will gain the knowledge that will ultimately impact the outcome of their techniques for limb preservation.

Peter A. Blume, DPM, FACFAS
Anesthesia and Orthopedics and Rehabilitation
Yale School of Medicine
New Haven, CT, USA

E-mail address:
peter.b@snet.net

Perioperative Management of the Patient with Diabetes Mellitus
Update and Overview

Stephen M. Schroeder, DPM

KEYWORDS

- Diabetes mellitus • Management • Glycemic control • Comorbidities

KEY POINTS

- Some of the primary factors that put diabetic patients at higher risk are poor glycemic control, the existence of comorbidities, and failure to recognize the condition.
- Poor long-term and short-term blood sugar control has been shown to delay healing and increase the risk of postoperative infections throughout multiple specialties.
- Diabetic patients are often elderly with comorbidities including cardiovascular disease, impaired renal function, respiratory disease, and peripheral vascular disease. Diabetic surgical patients often present with one or more of these conditions and need to be properly addressed in order to proceed safely with the planned procedure.
- Proper perioperative management of diabetic patients starts by identifying those with the disease state. Of the estimated 25 million Americans with diabetes, 7 million (28%) do not know they have it and only become aware when a complication arises. It has been established by the American Diabetes Association that controlling perioperative blood sugars for orthopedic surgical patients can decrease mortality, reduce infection rates, and lead to shorter lengths of stay in the hospital.
- Perioperative management of diabetic patients centers on optimizing glycemic control and negotiating comorbidities to help reduce complications and obtain results on par with nondiabetics.
- Taking a team approach in managing these complex patients leads to improved outcomes and is now considered the standard of care.

INTRODUCTION

The incidence of diabetes continues to escalate in the United States and throughout the world. Diabetes has deleterious affects on multiple body systems and is the leading cause of blindness, end-stage renal disease, and nontraumatic amputations.[1] Peripheral neuropathy and vascular disease lead to lower extremity complications that correlate directly with higher morbidity and mortality. In addition, the sequelae

Disclosure: The author has nothing to disclose and no conflicts of interest to report.
Sports Medicine Oregon, 7300 Southwest Childs Road, Suite B, Tigard, OR 97224, USA
E-mail address: sschroeder@osma1.com

Clin Podiatr Med Surg 31 (2014) 1–10
http://dx.doi.org/10.1016/j.cpm.2013.10.002 **podiatric.theclinics.com**

of diabetes create complex scenarios that make treatment challenging. The disease is directly related to increased morbidity and length of stay in hospitals.[2] It is estimated that up to 25% of hospitalized Americans have diabetes. Surgical patients are estimated to stay in house 45% longer and have 5 times higher mortality than nondiabetic patients.[3]

Some of the primary factors that put diabetic patients at higher risk are poor glycemic control, the existence of comorbidities, and failure to recognize the condition. Poor long-term and short-term blood sugar control has been shown to delay healing and increase the risk of postoperative infections throughout multiple specialties.[4]

Diabetic patients are often elderly with comorbidities including cardiovascular disease, impaired renal function, respiratory disease, and peripheral vascular disease.[5] There is a 2-fold to 4-fold increase of cardiovascular disease in diabetic patients that may include hypertension, coronary artery disease, or stroke.[6] Diabetic surgical patients often present with one or more of these conditions and need to be properly addressed in order to proceed safely with the planned procedure.

There is a common misconception that surgery should not be performed on diabetic patients for fear of complications and poor outcomes. Although certain aspects of diabetes can predispose patients to potential perioperative complications, improved understanding of the disease process combined with newer technology, a team-oriented approach, and better anesthesia techniques makes surgery a less harrowing proposition. This article focuses on perioperative management of diabetic patients. It gives advice on ways to prepare patients during this time in order to optimize outcomes for elective and nonelective procedures.

PERIOPERATIVE ASSESSMENT

Proper perioperative management of diabetic patients starts by identifying those with the disease state. Patients who have established medical care with a primary care physician (PCP) are typically identified. However, there is an increasing number of people in the United States without medical insurance, who do not have proper access to a PCP, and who may have unrecognized and untreated diabetes. Of the estimated 25 million Americans with diabetes, 7 million (28%) do not know they have it and only become aware when a complication arises,[7] which is particularly problematic for patients requiring emergency surgery because hyperglycemia and other comorbidities cannot be properly managed before surgery, which may lead to increased complications.[8] Patients with undocumented but suspected diabetes should be worked up by checking serum glucose and glycosylated hemoglobin A1c (HbA1c) levels before surgery.

Identification of these patients is done with a thorough history and physical examination. The history should detail symptoms of cardiac, neurologic, peripheral vascular (peripheral vascular disease [PVD]), retinal, and renal disease. It is important that patients with cardiac disease, PVD, or renal disease get proper preoperative clearance from their PCP or particular specialist before undergoing elective surgery. Proper referrals should be made before moving forward if they are not established with a PCP or specialist. Box 1 and Tables 1 and 2 detail elements that should be included in the preoperative work-up.

PERIOPERATIVE MANAGEMENT
Cardiac Disease

The risk for cardiac events in foot and ankle surgery is typically considered to be low (<1%).[9] However, the mortality from heart disease in diabetic patients is 2 to 4 times higher than for nondiabetics. The risk of postoperative complications increases when

> **Box 1**
> **Elements that should be included in a preoperative physical examination**
>
> *Physical Examination*
>
> - Blood pressure
> - Thyroid palpation
> - Cardiac evaluation
> - Pulmonary evaluation
> - Abdominal palpation
> - Evaluation of peripheral pulses
> - Foot examination
> - Skin examination
> - Neurologic examination

there is a history of myocardial infarction, atrial fibrillation, or congestive heart failure.[10] It is important to work these patients up at the very least with an electrocardiogram (ECG). Any abnormality or history of cardiac issues warrants a cardiology referral for further evaluation and clearance before surgery. The goal is to identify potential problems that may lead to perioperative cardiac events and then minimize those risks.

Further cardiac work-up begins with an evaluation of functional capacity. Laboratory tests can be obtained to identify any abnormal cardiac markers. Noninvasive testing is also common and may include ECG, echocardiography assessing left ventricular function, chemical stress testing, and exercise stress testing. When necessary, coronary angiography may be performed to complete the work-up.

Once potential problems are identified, steps can be taken to minimize risk and optimize outcomes. Pharmacologic risk reduction strategies may include β-blockers, nitrates, statins, angiotensin-converting enzyme (ACE) inhibitors, calcium channel blockers, diuretics, aspirin, or anticoagulation therapy. Perioperative β-blocker therapy has been shown to decrease the incidence of postoperative myocardial ischemia and infarction, and should be considered in all diabetics undergoing surgery. More advanced procedures such as percutaneous intracoronary intervention or coronary artery bypass grafting are occasionally recommended to optimize perioperative success. Suggestions may also me given to monitor patients in the hospital with telemetry if there is concern for acute cardiac events (**Table 3**).[11]

Renal Disease

Kidney disease is a common complication of diabetes and affects as many as 50% of this population. Diabetic nephropathy is the leading cause of kidney disease in the United States and is responsible for 30% to 40% of all end-stage renal disease (ESRD). There is a high associated morbidity and mortality and it can lead to significant perioperative complications including infections, delayed healing or nonhealing of surgical sites, acute renal failure, hyperkalemia, and volume overload.[13]

These patients have impaired synthetic function causing a decrease in erythropoietin and active vitamin D_3 production, as well as limited potassium, salt, water, and acid excretion. Care is needed to prevent drugs excreted through the renal route accumulating to toxic levels. Platelet dysfunction can also occur, leading to excessive intraoperative bleeding. In addition, up to 50% of patients with renal disease have reduced renal blood flow with the administration of general anesthesia.

Table 1
Elements that should be included in a preoperative history

History Questionnaire	Examples
Systemic symptoms of diabetes	Polyuria Polydipsia Blurred vision
Family history	Diabetes Cardiac disease Anesthesia complications
Social history	Dietary habits History of malnutrition Tobacco use Alcohol use Controlled substance use
Current diabetes management	Medications Diet Exercise Glucose monitoring results
History of acute diabetic complications	Ketoacidosis Hypoglycemia Acute renal failure
History of infections	Skin Feet Dentition Genitourinary system
History of vascular complications	Deep vein thrombosis Pulmonary Embolism (PE) Cerebrovascular events
History of cardiac disease complications	Severe hypertension Atrial fibrillation Unstable angina Aortic stenosis Congestive heart failure Myocardial infarction Stroke
Current medications	Corticosteroids Hypertensive medications Cholesterol-reducing medications Diuretics Diabetic medications Insulin
Risk factors for atherosclerosis	Smoking Hypertension Obesity Dyslipidemia Family history of atherosclerosis

Evaluation by a nephrologist before surgery is recommended in order to optimize renal function and minimize complications. A basic metabolic panel (BMP) is ordered to assess renal function and electrolyte levels. Most patients can be managed medically but some may require perioperative dialysis depending on the type of surgery and severity of the disease. Diabetic patients with kidney disease often have

Table 2
Additional testing that should be considered during the work-up

Additional Tests	Useful Information
Electrocardiogram	Identifies potential cardiac disorders
Laboratory Tests	
Basic metabolic panel	Measures serum glucose level, gives electrolyte levels, and measures renal function
HbA1C	Identifies the average plasma glucose concentration over several months
Complete blood count	Measures white blood cell count, which can be an indicator of infection, hemoglobin, hematocrit, and platelet count
C-reactive protein	Inflammatory marker that is often increased in the presence of bone infection
Erythrocyte sedimentation rate	Inflammatory marker

Table 3
Major perioperative complications in diabetic patients with cardiac disease

Major Complication	Preventative Therapy
Myocardial infarction	Evaluate for myocardial ischemia Use perioperative β-blockers Encourage strict glycemic control Lipid-reducing therapy Use aspirin or other antiplatelet medications Maintain blood pressure <130/80 mm Hg
Stroke[12]	Use perioperative β-blockers Use perioperative ACE inhibitors Strict glycemic control Use aspirin or other antiplatelet medications Lipid-reducing therapy

Table 4
Major perioperative complications in diabetic patients with renal disease

Major Complication	Preventative Therapy
Renal insufficiency	Optimize blood pressure control Optimize glycemic control Use perioperative ACE inhibitors Minimize use of nephrotoxic agents Limit protein intake to 0.8 g/kg/d

Table 5
Guideline for perioperative dose management of oral hypoglycemic medications on the day of surgery

Medication	AM Surgery	PM Surgery
Acarbose	Hold AM dose if NPO	Give AM dose if eating breakfast
Meglitinide	Hold AM dose if NPO	Give AM dose if eating breakfast
Metformin	Take normal dose	Take normal dose
Sulfonylurea	Hold AM dose if NPO	Hold AM and PM dose
Pioglitazone	Take normal dose	Take normal dose
DPP-4 inhibitor	Omit on day of surgery	Omit on day of surgery
GLP-1 analogue	Omit on day of surgery	Omit on day of surgery

Abbreviations: DPP-4, dipeptidyl peptidase 4; GLP-1, glucagonlike peptide 1; NPO, nil by mouth.
Data from American Diabetes Association. All about diabetes. Available at: http://www.diabetes.org/about-diabetes.jsp. Accessed February 26, 2013.

Table 6
Guideline for perioperative dose management of insulin on the day of surgery (always check serum glucose on admission)

Insulin	AM Surgery	PM Surgery
Once-a-day AM dose • Lantus • Humulin I	Take normal AM dose	Take normal AM dose
Once-a-day PM dose • Lantus • Humulin I	Take normal PM dose if eating	Take normal PM dose if eating
Twice-a-day dosing • Novomix 30 • Humulin M3 • Humalog Mix 25 • Humalog Mix 50 • Lantus	Take half the normal AM dose Take normal PM dose if eating	Take half the normal AM dose Take normal PM dose if eating
Twice a day, short acting • Novorapid • Humulin S	Calculate the total dose of both morning insulins and give half as intermediate acting only in the morning	Calculate the total dose of both morning insulins and give half as intermediate acting only in the morning
Intermediate acting • Humulin I • Insuman	Take normal PM dose if eating	Take normal PM dose if eating
3, 4, or 5 doses per day	Basal bolus regimens: Hold short-acting AM and lunchtime doses Take the normal basal dose Premixed AM insulin: Take half the normal AM dose Hold lunchtime dose	Take normal AM dose

Data from American Diabetes Association. All about diabetes. Available at: http://www.diabetes.org/about-diabetes.jsp. Accessed February 26, 2013.

associated cardiac disease. β-Blocker therapy has been shown to reduce perioperative complication and should also be considered. Patients with ESRD on hemodialysis ideally undergo therapy before surgery in order to reduce the risk of excessive bleeding, volume overload, and hyperkalemia. This therapy should be done within 24 hours of the procedure for optimal results (**Table 4**).[14]

Glucose Control

The next step in perioperative management of the diabetic patient is optimizing serum glucose levels. Increased serum glucose hinders proper leukocyte function, impairing chemotaxis and phagocyte activity. It has been suggested that this leads to an increase in infections in diabetics, accounting for 66% of postoperative complications and 25% of perioperative deaths.[15] The key to successfully achieving glucose control is frequent serum glucose monitoring and medication adjustments based on the findings.[16]

Surgery creates certain stresses on the body, leading to an increase in secretion of catabolic hormones such as epinephrine, glucocorticoids, and growth hormone, all of which increase blood glucose concentrations. Secretion of anabolic hormones, including insulin, are inhibited. This inhibition creates insulin resistance after surgery and functional insulin insufficiency. The effect is most profound in major and emergency surgery.[17] Type I diabetics have no capacity to secrete insulin and are unable to respond to the increased demand during surgery. Type II diabetics have a reduced

---

Table 7
Example of a standard insulin sliding scale order often used after surgery or when patients are transitioning off, or back onto, their normal insulin regimens

Regular insulin (eg, Humulin-R) sliding scale, standard orders. Recommended indications:
- As a supplement to a patient's usual diabetes medications (long-acting insulin or oral agents) to treat uncontrolled high blood sugars
- For short-term use (24–48 h) in a patient admitted with an unknown insulin requirement Regimens:
- Low-dose scale: suggested starting point for thin and elderly, or those being initiated on total parenteral nutrition
- Moderate-dose scale: suggested starting point for average patient
- High-dose scale: suggested for patients with infections or those receiving therapy with high-dose corticosteroids

Blood Sugar (mg/dL)	Low-dose Scale	Moderate-dose Scale	High-dose Scale	Patient-specific Scale
<70	Initiate hypoglycemia protocol	Initiate hypoglycemia protocol	Initiate hypoglycemia protocol	Initiate hypoglycemia protocol
70–130	0 units	0 units	0 units	____ units
131–180	2 units	4 units	8 units	____ units
181–240	4 units	8 units	12 units	____ units
241–300	6 units	10 units	16 units	____ units
301–350	8 units	12 units	20 units	____ units
351–400	10 units	16 units	24 units	____ units
>400	12 units and call MD	20 units and call MD	28 units and call MD	____ units and call MD

Abbreviation: MD, Doctor of Medicine.

ability to respond to demand because they are insulin resistant and have a low reserve.

The inhalation agents used in anesthesia can also suppress insulin secretion and lead to abnormal glucose regulation and hyperglycemia.[18] Local peripheral nerve blocks may mitigate this response and should be considered when appropriate.

The benefits of strict perioperative insulin regulation have been well documented and this is now the standard of care for diabetic surgery.[19] With stricter control there is also a risk for developing hypoglycemia. The goal is to balance the benefits of tight glycemic control with the potential for hypoglycemia.

There is still some debate as to the optimal glycemic level. Most institutions have deployed dedicated multidisciplinary glycemic control teams with set guidelines to manage these patients during their hospital stays both before and after surgery. These teams have been shown to reduce the length of stay for patients with diabetes and should always be used when doing inpatient diabetic surgery.[20]

A multidisciplinary team approach should also be taken when performing elective outpatient diabetic surgery. Serum glucose levels and HbA1c levels should be evaluated. HbA1c is an indicator for how well (or poorly) blood sugars have been managed over several months. Levels of 6% or less are optimum but 6% to 8% is generally considered safe for avoiding major postoperative complications. An increased

Table 8
Key perioperative management points for foot and ankle surgeons to improve outcomes in diabetic surgical patients

Key Point	Example
Establish realistic surgical outcome expectations with the patient	Diabetes brings the possibility of higher surgical complications Possibility of a slower recovery than normal It is importance to comply with instructions Strict elevation and limited activity for a period of time after surgery
Create an understanding of what the patient can do to reduce postoperative complications	Control hyperglycemia before and after surgery Stop smoking Comply with instructions Take medications as directed
Give clear instructions for oral hypoglycemic medications and/or insulin on the day of surgery	See **Tables 5–7**
Understand the patient's level of glycemic control	Proper history BMP for serum glucose HbA1c for long-term control
Recognize the potential for cardiac disease in an undiagnosed patient	Smoking Overweight Lower extremity edema Family history ECG findings
Recognize the potential for renal disease in an undiagnosed patient	BMP Fluid pretension Lower extremity edema
Get help when appropriate	Seek preoperative clearance Glycemic control team consult

HbA1c has been associated with poorer surgical outcomes whether or not diabetes has been diagnosed.[21] Elective surgery should be delayed for several months in patients with HbA1c levels higher than 8% in order to optimize control and reduce risk for complications. Before surgery, consultation with the patient's PCP or endocrinologist is advised to help optimize glucose control.

It has been established by the American Diabetes Association that controlling perioperative blood sugars for orthopedic surgical patients can decrease mortality, reduce infection rates, and lead to shorter lengths of stay in the hospital. The recommended fasting blood glucose target for most surgical patients is 90 to 126 mg/dL. The recommended random blood glucose target is less than 200 mg/dL.[7] Depending on the situation and severity of disease, perioperative blood sugar can be managed by oral agents, insulin therapy, insulin sliding scales, or intravenous (IV) insulin infusion. **Tables 5** and **6** give guidelines for proper oral medication and insulin dosage on the day of surgery. **Table 7** shows an example of a standard insulin sliding scale often used after surgery or when patients are transitioning off, or back onto, their normal insulin regimens.

SUMMARY

Perioperative management of diabetic patients centers on optimizing glycemic control and negotiating comorbidities to help reduce complications and obtain results on par with nondiabetics. These goals are usually achievable in the elective surgical setting, but they can be more difficult to control in urgent or emergent situations. Understanding and recognizing the comorbidities associated with diabetes is imperative for optimizing outcomes. Regulating hyperglycemia can reduce morbidity, mortality, and postoperative infections.[4] This is accomplished using oral agents, insulin therapy, insulin sliding scales, or IV insulin infusion. Understanding the effects of cardiac and renal disease is also important when trying to ensure a good outcome.[6] Taking a team approach in managing these complex patients leads to improved outcomes and is now considered the standard of care (**Table 8**).

REFERENCES

1. Hoogwerf BJ, Sferra J, Donley BG. Diabetes mellitus–overview. Foot Ankle Clin 2006;11:703–15.
2. Moghissi ES, Korytkowski MT, DiNardo M, et al. American Association of Clinical Endocrinologists and American Diabetic Association consensus statement on inpatient glycemic control. Diabetes Care 2009;32:1119–31.
3. Hall GM, Page SR. Diabetes and surgery. In: Page SR, Hall GM, editors. Emergency and hospital management. London: BMJ Publishing; 1999.
4. Frisch A, Chandra P, Smiley D, et al. Prevalence and clinical outcome of hyperglycemia in the perioperative period in noncardiac surgery. Diabetes Care 2010;33: 1783–8.
5. Cuthbertson BH, Amiri AR, Croal BL, et al. Utility of B-type natriuretic peptide in predicting medium-term mortality in patients undergoing major non-cardiac surgery. Am J Cardiol 2007;100:1310–3.
6. Stamler J, Vaccaro O, Neaton JD, et al. Diabetes, other risk factors, and 12-yr cardiovascular mortality for men screened in the multiple risk factor intervention trial. Diabetes Care 1993;16:434–44.
7. American Diabetes Association. All about diabetes. Available at: http://www. diabetes.org/about-diabetes.jsp. Accessed February 26, 2013.

8. Levetan CS, Passaro M, Jabloski K, et al. Unrecognized diabetes among hospitalized patients. Diabetes Care 1998;21:246–9.
9. Boersma E, Kertai MD, Schouten O, et al. Perioperative cardiovascular mortality in noncardiac surgery: validation of the Lee cardiac risk index. Am J Med 2005; 118:1134–41.
10. Kumar R, McKinney WP, Raj G, et al. Adverse cardiac events after surgery: assessing risk in a veteran population. J Gen Intern Med 2001;16:507–18.
11. Poldermans D, Bax JJ, Boersma E, et al. Guidelines for pre-operative cardiac risk assessment and perioperative cardiac management in non-cardiac surgery. Eur Heart J 2009;30(22):2769–812.
12. Adams HP Jr, del Zoppo G, Alberts MJ, et al. Guidelines for the early management of adults with ischemic stroke: a guideline from the American Heart Association/American Stroke Association Stroke Council, Clinical Cardiology Council, Cardiovascular Radiology and Intervention Council, and the Atherosclerotic Peripheral Vascular Disease and Quality of Care Outcomes in Research Interdisciplinary Working Groups: the American Academy of Neurology affirms the value of this guideline as an educational tool for neurologists. Stroke 2007;38(5): 1655–711.
13. de Boer IH, Rue TC, Hall YN, et al. Temporal trends in the prevalence of diabetic kidney disease in the United States. JAMA 2011;305(24):2532–9.
14. Trainor D, Borthwick E, Ferguson A. Perioperative management of the hemodialysis patient. Semin Dial 2011;24(3):314–26.
15. Loh-Trivedi M. Perioperative management of the diabetic patient. Medscape Online Journal. 2013. Available at: www.emedicine.medscape.com/article/284451. Accessed June 10, 2013.
16. Marks JB. Perioperative management of diabetes. Am Fam Physician 2003;67(1): 93–100.
17. Desborough JP. The stress response to trauma and surgery. Br J Anaesth 2000; 85:109–17.
18. McAnulty GR, Robertshaw HJ, Hall GM. Anaesthetic management of patients with diabetes mellitus. Br J Anaesth 2000;85(1):80–90.
19. Van den Berghe G, Wilmer A, Hermans G, et al. Intensive insulin therapy in the medical ICU. N Engl J Med 2006;354(5):449–61.
20. Flanagan D, Moore E, Baker S, et al. Diabetes care in hospital: the impact of a dedicated inpatient care team. Diabet Med 2008;25:147–51.
21. O'Sullivan CJ, Hynes N, Mahendran B, et al. Hemoglobin A1c (HbA1c) in non-diabetic and diabetic vascular patients: is HbA1c an independent risk factor and predictor of adverse outcome? Eur J Vasc Endovasc Surg 2006;32:188–97.

Diabetes Mellitus and Peripheral Vascular Disease
Diagnosis and Management

Jason A. Chin, MD, Bauer E. Sumpio, MD*

KEYWORDS

- Diabetes mellitus • Peripheral artery disease • PAD • Peripheral vascular disease

KEY POINTS

- Diabetes and peripheral artery disease (PAD) are both coronary heart disease equivalents and the pathologic cardiovascular processes of one may impact and augment that of the other.
- Be alert for atypical presentations of PAD, as classic symptoms, such as claudication and physical examination findings, may be altered by concurrent presence of diabetes.
- Many noninvasive and imaging studies are available; however, computed tomography angiography is the new standard in assessing PAD and planning for surgical or endovascular intervention.
- Medical management of both diseases includes goal HbA1c lower than 7.0%, blood pressure lower than 130/80, low density lipoprotein lower than 70 mg/dL, and treatment with aspirin and possibly clopidogrel.
- Surgical bypass to revascularize the lower extremities generally requires fewer reinterventions than endovascular therapies, although limb salvage rates appear similar, and both modalities should attempt to restore straight-line pulsatile flow to the foot.

INTRODUCTION: NATURE OF THE PROBLEM

Taken together, diabetes mellitus (DM) and peripheral artery disease (PAD) represent 2 of the fastest growing and most challenging medical-surgical diseases facing the world today. As coronary heart disease risk equivalents, they put patients at significant risk for cardiovascular events and mortality in addition to their other common morbidities, including limb loss. Epidemiologically, they have a quickly growing prevalence in not just developed nations but also developing nations. Acting on peripheral vasculature together, they often present difficult treatment choices from both medical and surgical standpoints. This review provides a brief overview of these disease entities,

Section of Vascular Surgery, Department of Surgery, Yale University School of Medicine, 333 Cedar Street, BB 204, New Haven, CT 06510, USA
* Corresponding author.
E-mail address: bauer.sumpio@yale.edu

Clin Podiatr Med Surg 31 (2014) 11–26
http://dx.doi.org/10.1016/j.cpm.2013.09.001
0891-8422/14/$ – see front matter © 2014 Elsevier Inc. All rights reserved.

as well as options for their treatment both medically and surgically. Particular attention is paid to the lower extremities of patients with both diseases, as the diagnosis and management in these situations can provide a unique set of challenges.

Epidemiology

The prevalence of DM has risen in the United States at an alarming rate, particularly type 2. Recent Centers for Disease Control and Prevention estimates of the diagnosed prevalence puts 7.8% of the American population with DM, nearly double the prevalence of 4.9% in 1990.[1] This correlates with rising obesity in Americans, now present in 20% of adults. In terms of absolute numbers, 24 million American adults are diabetic in addition to 57 million prediabetic individuals. A rising incidence is noted in the developing world, including China, which has a 1% prevalence of DM but is projected to rise to 8% to 10%.[2]

With regard to PAD, there is an estimated worldwide prevalence of almost 10%, with 15% to 20% of people older than 70 years affected.[3,4] Critical limb ischemia, PAD's most severe manifestation, has an annual incidence of approximately 500 to 1000 per million.[5]

Examining these 2 together, DM doubles the likelihood of developing PAD, and a 1% increase in HbA1c is associated with a 26% increase in risk of developing PAD.[6,7] Furthermore, PAD patients with diabetes are 5–10 times more likely to progress to major amputation compared to PAD patients without diabetes.[8] Despite these morbid statistics, the true prevalence of PAD in diabetic patients has been somewhat difficult to determine, as the reported symptoms and objective findings are often not typical of each of the diseases alone. Many patients may be asymptomatic and others may have an atypical pain pattern due to peripheral neuropathy. The PARTNERS study by general practitioners in diabetic patients older than 50 years used ankle-brachial indexes (ABIs) to diagnose PAD in 29% of patients.[2] Likewise, 50% of patients with diabetic foot ulcers have PAD.[5]

Although exact statistics tend to vary across different studies and populations, none would dispute the association between DM and PAD. Full treatment of one disease will require awareness and optimization of the other.

Pathologic Basis

Diabetes mellitus

The pathophysiology of DM is a highly complex system of both innate and environmental factors that is beyond the scope of this discussion. Briefly, however, DM is classically broken down into type 1 and type 2. Type 1 DM is generally thought of as a chronic autoimmune disease.[9] Indeed, the common pathologic finding is lymphocytic infiltration of the pancreatic islets, with destruction of insulin-secreting beta cells. Of individuals with type 1 DM, 90% are known to have autoantibodies against islets cells, insulin, or glutamic acid decarboxylase; however, the mechanism of these antibodies as cause or effect of type 1 DM remains to be elucidated. As far as its pathogenesis, current models describe an environmental factor triggering an autoimmune response in susceptible patients, which over years leads to destruction of pancreatic beta cells and thereby decreased insulin secretion. Once 80% to 90% of these cells are lost, hyperglycemia may develop and patients will present themselves: 20% with fulminant diabetic ketoacidosis.[2] Over the following months, complete destruction of beta cells renders these patients insulin-dependent.

Type 2 DM, in contrast, is a more heterogeneous and more common entity characterized by insulin resistance. Its association with obesity is well described and accounts for the currently increasing prevalence in young patients in whom obesity rates are also increasing. Although no specific gene can account for the disease, genetics plays a strong role, as evidenced by a strong family history in diabetic patients and nearly 100% concordance in identical twins. Insulin resistance has been found to be far greatest over skeletal muscle beds in glucose extraction studies comparing different organ beds, emphasizing the need for exercise in treating type 2 DM.[2] Interestingly, although insulin resistance has been thought to be the primary mediator of hyperglycemia, impaired insulin secretion associated with hyperglycemia may play a role as well. A "Starling curve" of insulin secretion has been described for varying levels of blood glucose wherein the highest levels of insulin responsiveness may be seen at approximately 120 mg/dL and then taper significantly for glucose levels above and below that. Thus, hyperglycemia may impair insulin secretion and action.[10]

PAD in DM

As noted previously, patients with PAD and DM are more likely to progress to more severe stages of disease more quickly. Multiple studies have made attempts to explain this pathophysiology in terms of vessel wall, cell, and inflammatory dysfunction. Although verging on overly simplistic, PAD is inflammatory damage to the vessel wall due to endothelial cell dysfunction resulting in stenosis and occlusion. A common outcome for most mediators of endothelial dysfunction in DM is decreased nitric oxide (NO) bioavailability. NO normally stimulates vasodilation while limiting inflammation, vascular smooth cell migration and proliferation, and platelet activation, which all contribute to the progression of arterial wall damage, stenosis, and occlusion. Hyperglycemia blocks endothelial NO synthase (eNOS) and increases reactive oxygen species, causing wall damage.[11] Insulin resistance also leads to increased free fatty acid levels, which can cause oxidative damage and activate proinflammatory pathways, such as the mitogen-activated protein kinase pathway.[12] It should also be noted that the inflammatory marker C-reactive protein (CRP), a risk factor for PAD, is elevated in patients with DM.[13] CRP is known to promote apoptosis of endothelial cells as well cause further vascular dysfunction through stimulating production of tissue factor and chemotactic substances, leukocyte adhesion, and inhibiting eNOS.

The molecular pathways of PAD and DM represent complex processes, but it is worth understanding their synergism and its implications for accelerated disease progression when the 2 diseases present simultaneously.

PATIENT HISTORY

DM may present with a variety of symptoms at varying stages of the disease and differently between patients with type 1 and type 2. The full clinical presentation of DM is not discussed here, but it suffices to say that patients will often be referred to podiatric and vascular surgery specialists with a preexisting diagnosis of DM. Current American Diabetes Association (ADA) expert consensus for diagnosis of DM are one of any of the following[14]:

- Symptoms and random blood glucose level greater than 200 mg/dL
- HbA1c greater than 6.5%
- Fasting blood glucose level greater than 126 mg/dL on 2 separate occasions
- Two-hour blood glucose level greater than 200 mg/dL after a 75-g oral glucose load

PAD typically presents with intermittent claudication: aching muscle pain triggered by exercise and relieved by rest. The location of this pain will occur distal to the area of arterial stenosis or occlusion; stenosis in the iliac arteries, femoral arteries, and tibioperoneal arteries will cause pain in the buttock/thigh, calf, and foot, respectively.

In contrast, patients with both PAD and DM may have a more atypical clinical picture. Although lower extremity arterial stenosis usually associated with PAD is focal and most commonly in the superficial femoral artery causing calf pain, patients with DM will often have diffuse and severe disease more commonly involving the tibial arteries with high prevalence of long occlusions.[15] This can be thought to cause more pain in the foot; however, the additional peripheral neuropathy associated with DM can even make these patients asymptomatic. One should be observant of more subtle findings, including leg fatigue and progressively slowing ambulation. Collateral formation is also reduced in patients with DM, making them more susceptible to severe and acute ischemia.[16] This may present with deep duskiness and pain of the extremity caused by atherosclerotic plaque rupture or in situ thrombosis of a vessel. Indeed, one study showed the incidence of acute thrombosis in diabetic patients with PAD was 35% with a 21% major amputation compared with 19% and 3%, respectively, in nondiabetic patients with PAD.[17] In the setting of this cloudy clinical picture, it is also important to realize usual indirect measures of lower extremity blood pressures, such as ABIs, can be rendered unreliable by the characteristic medial sclerosis, calcification of the tunica media causing rigid arteries, of DM compared with the more usual intimal process of nondiabetic atherosclerosis.[18]

Podiatric and vascular specialists must be especially vigilant for these atypical presentations of PAD in diabetic patients, as the data note the consequences of a missed diagnosis can be sudden and dire.

PHYSICAL EXAMINATION

Although specialist-referred patients may often present with focal complaints, such as a foot ulcer or calf pain, it is essential to perform a comprehensive physical examination, as both DM and PAD are systemic processes that may be revealed by findings elsewhere in the body. Vital signs of heart rate, respiratory rate, oxygen saturation, blood pressure, and temperature are essential. Asymmetric blood pressure in the upper extremities may point to entities such as subclavian stenosis that would provide further reason to suspect lower extremity disease. Fever, tachycardia, and tachypnea may suggest evolving sepsis in an otherwise asymptomatic foot ulcer.

Vascular Examination

Although many practitioners may limit their vascular examination to palpation of pedal pulses, assessment of all peripheral pulses is essential for diagnosing PAD, including bilateral carotid (these should be first auscultated for bruits), brachial, radial, femoral, popliteal, dorsalis pedis, and posterior tibial arteries. In addition to allowing assessment of multilevel arterial disease, palpation of these pulses, particularly the femoral pulses, may be important in planning for different endovascular or surgical intervention options where access or bypass sites might be precluded by local disease. Patients with more severe disease often have nonpalpable pulses; therefore, a handheld Doppler evaluation of flow signals is also essential. The quality of the signals should be graded as follows:

- Triphasic: normal arterial flow and usually associated with a palpable pulse
- Biphasic: mild to moderate PAD
- Monophasic or absent: severe PAD

Other qualities that can be used to assess vascular health in an extremity include skin and nail changes. Diminished blood flow may equate to diminished nutritional supply to the skin, which may be manifested as dry, shiny, and hairless skin. Nails may also become brittle and rigid. One pertinent finding in lower extremities with chronic arterial ischemia is elevation pallor and dependent rubor. This is due to the loss of the venoarteriolar reflex. As ischemia progresses, venules and arterioles dilate to compensate for the ischemia, whereas they would normally constrict in the dependent position. This leads to a pale white appearance when the limb is elevated and blood flows out of these small vessels and a deep purple or red in the dependent position when blood pools.[19] Skin temperature may be compared from one extremity to another to help assess perfusion, although this should take into account the ambient temperature during the examination and other confounding factors.

Ulcer Examination

Particular attention should be paid to any ulcers in patients with PAD and DM, given the morbid statistics of major limb amputation noted previously. Arterial disease in a diabetic patient compounds the already increased risk of ulcer formation and progression in diabetic individuals. If their diabetic neuropathy is severe, patients may present with ulcers unknowingly, which mandates a thorough physical examination, especially of all aspects of the patient's feet. Ulcerations secondary to ischemia are often on the tips of digits and in the interdigital spaces, whereas neuropathic ulcers usually occur over the heel or metatarsal head pressure points on the plantar surface of the foot. These findings may help contribute to suspicion of one process or the other, but ultimately, a vascular examination should be performed to assess for any detriments to healing potential whether the ulcer is ischemic, neuropathic, or both.

Ulcer characteristics, such as size, depth, appearance, presence of bleeding, and granulation tissue, should be documented to assist in evaluating progression over time. It is also important to probe ulcers with a cotton-tip probe or other similar instrument to clarify the presence of sinus tracts and undermining. Superficial fibrotic tissue that may appear intact can easily break down with minimal force on probing. This is also important to establish the diagnosis of osteomyelitis, should the probe be able to be extended down to bone. One study showed a positive probe-to-bone test has 98% sensitivity, 78% specificity, 95% positive predictive value, and 91% negative predictive value for diagnosing osteomyelitis when compared with standard bone histology and culture.[20] In the setting of arterial insufficiency and infection, such ulcers may be particularly difficult to heal. A positive test should be added with other findings when considering initiation of treatment, but should at least trigger further imaging evaluations if not starting treatment.

IMAGING AND ADDITIONAL TESTING
Noninvasive Studies

If the diagnosis of PAD is in doubt or if the diagnosis is already established, further noninvasive testing is valuable for assessing the severity of arterial insufficiency. First among these tests is the ABI. This is derived first by determining the systolic blood pressure in both brachial arteries and then in both of each the dorsalis pedis and posterior tibial arteries. It can then be calculated for each lower extremity and interpreted as in **Table 1**.

In patients with DM, the ABI can be less reliable, as noted previously, due to false elevations secondary to vessel calcification and noncompressibility. Although it does not accurately gauge lower extremity perfusion, an ABI greater than 1.3 is associated with increased cardiovascular event rates.[21] A normal or subnormal ABI in a diabetic patient, however, should prompt health care providers to consider the possibility of even worse vascular disease than the value would imply in nondiabetic patients.

Table 1 ABI = Highest ankle pressure (dorsalis pedis or posterior tibial) in a leg/Highest arm pressure (right or left)	
ABI	**Interpretation**
>1.3	False elevation; heavy vessel calcification
0.9–1.3	Normal
0.5–0.9	Peripheral artery disease; associated with intermittent claudication
<0.5	Critical limb ischemia; associated with ulceration and rest pain

Abbreviation: ABI, ankle-brachial index.

Pulse volume recordings (PVRs) seen in **Fig. 1** can also be obtained relatively easily using multiple pneumatic cuffs and pressure sensors at different levels on each leg. The waveforms at each level can then be interpreted as triphasic, biphasic, monophasic, or flat, as might be done with listening to Doppler signals or also obtaining waveforms using Doppler spectral analysis.

Having said that ABIs may be less reliable in diabetic patients, other noninvasive means can be used to assess disease severity and ulcer healing potential if present. Toe pressures should be measured and can more reliably assess forefoot circulation, as arteries at this level tend to be spared from atherosclerotic processes. Toe pressure lower than 55 mm Hg or toe-brachial index less than 0.7 has been associated with PAD, and toe pressures lower than 30 mm Hg usually indicate that a wound is unlikely to heal on that extremity.[6,21]

A variety of other noninvasive perfusion tests are in development and have undergone study for assessing wound healing, including such modalities as transcutaneous partial pressure of oxygen and hyperspectral imaging. However, variable accuracy is reported with these technologies, and edema, inflammation, and infection can all detract from their reliability. Ultimately, perfusion is only one factor assessing the healing potential of a wound, and consideration must be taken of other elements, such as active infection, edema, optimal wound care, hygiene, and risk factors such as smoking.

Many more detailed and costly imaging modalities are available to assess arterial circulation when physical examination and noninvasive tests leave questions.

Ultrasound

Duplex ultrasound is a fast, noninvasive, cost-effective method evaluating blood flow throughout the body. It can be easily performed in an outpatient or inpatient setting, although a skilled vascular ultrasound technologist is required for accurate results. Current devices can display imaging information with spectral waveforms and color flow maps seen in **Fig. 2**, both of which are important in deriving necessary physiologic information. It is important to note that tibial arteries are more difficult to assess compared with more proximal vessels, as it is at this level that PAD predominates in diabetic patients.[22] Sensitivities for detecting lesions with more than 50% reduction in diameter range from 89% in iliac arteries to 69% in popliteal arteries. Sensitivities for interruption of patency are up to 90% in the anterior and posterior tibial arteries and 82% in the peroneal artery.[23] Bowel gas, edema, skin ulceration, and vessel calcification can all limit the accuracy of ultrasound in the imaging of PAD.

Ultrasound remains as yet too involved and costly to replace the simple physical and noninvasive examinations noted previously; however, it serves as an important rapidly acquired imaging modality when noninvasive tests are inadequate but the

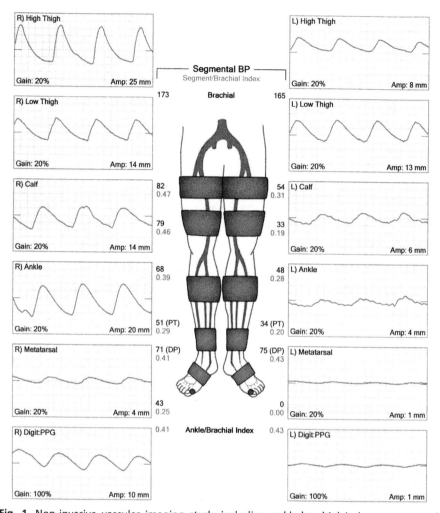

Fig. 1. Non-invasive vascular imaging study including ankle-brachial indexes, segmental pressures, and pulse volume recording (PVR) waveforms. Here the segmental pressures and indexes are higher on the right lower extremity at all levels compared to the left except for the dorsalis pedis artery. Biphasic PVR waveforms are seen at all levels on the right lower extremity. The left lower extremity has biphasic waveforms at the high thigh and low thigh, which then become blunted from the level of the calf down. This could indicate stenosis in the left superficial femoral artery or popliteal artery.

costs and other aspects of computed tomography, magnetic resonance imaging, and angiography, such as contrast and radiation, may be prohibitive. Ultrasound also serves as important follow-up and surveillance study after revascularization interventions have been performed. Graft and native vessels can be monitored on an outpatient basis, which can lead to greater long-term patency.[24]

Computed Tomography Angiography

Computed tomography angiography (CTA) seen in **Fig. 3** has rapidly become a new standard in the imaging of PAD with the introduction of increasing multidetector

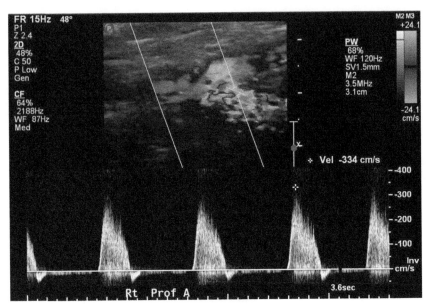

Fig. 2. Duplex ultrasound of the right profunda femoris and superficial femoral artery. The color flow ultrasound is seen in the upper part of the image and Doppler spectral waveforms are seen in the lower part. The Doppler waveforms here are biphasic.

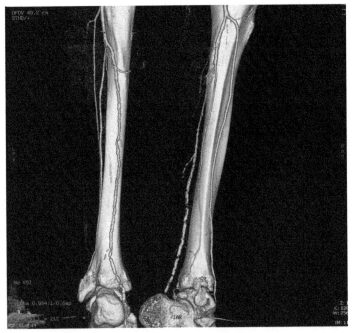

Fig. 3. 3D reconstruction of a CTA of bilateral lower extremities. This can depict intraluminal flow of contrast as well as vessel wall abnormalities and calcification. Bilateral posterior tibial arteries in this patient are severely calcified. This can be seen as the irregular, discontinuous densities in the distribution of the vessels. This is in contrast to the patent right anterior tibial artery which is the right-most vessel in the image.

scanners. Now up to 128-row scanners are available routinely. The introduction of the 64-row detector and delayed peripheral scan contrast protocols have overcome many of the limitations in imaging smaller and more heavily calcified tibial vessels in diabetic patients.[22] Compared with conventional digital subtraction angiography (DSA), CTA has near comparable accuracy for detecting stenosis of more than 50%. Reported sensitivities and specificities are 92% to 95% and 93% to 96%, respectively.[25,26] Another advantage of CTA compared with luminal imaging modalities, like magnetic resonance angiography (MRA) and DSA, include its ability to evaluate the vessel wall and atherosclerotic lesions for plaque characteristics, ulceration, calcification, and thrombus. CTA images should be reviewed with caution, however, as contrast may often be confused with diffusely and severely calcified vessel wall and vice versa. Other limitations include metal implants in the region of interest causing artifact, as well as the use of ionizing radiation and nephrotoxic contrast agents.[21]

MRA

MRA is another less invasive imaging study that has become more prevalent as the technology and relevant gadolinium contrast imaging protocols have evolved. The sensitivity and specificity for detecting hemodynamically significant lesions have both been reported up to 94% for peripheral arteries using MRA.[27] Of note, venous contamination can be problematic and reduce accuracy in tibial-level vessels, especially for patients with critical limb ischemia and diabetic foot ulcers.[22] Time-resolved imaging and other newer imaging protocols can help reduce this contamination and improve accuracy. MRA has the added advantage over CTA in not using ionizing radiation and the contrast agents are less nephrotoxic.

Compared with CTA, however, MRA generally suffers from poor spatial resolution and does not as readily provide information regarding the vessel, calcification, and plaque characteristics. Other important disadvantages remain its high cost compared with all other modalities and long imaging times, often longer than 60 minutes, which many patients cannot tolerate. Metal implants, such as pacemakers, defibrillators, and certain stents and aneurysm clips, may exclude patients from study. Most centers also will not image patients with glomerular filtration rate less than 30 mL per minute due to reports of nephrogenic systemic fibrosis.

DSA

DSA remains the gold standard of all imaging modalities for assessing the accuracy of other technologies, as it allows the highest spatial resolution of any imaging study. Its other main advantage is offering the opportunity to intervene on any discovered lesions using endovascular techniques that will be described later in this article. Despite this, it has become predominantly an interventional modality since the advent of the previously described imaging options. It is an invasive study requiring direct arterial puncture with all the complications associated with that, including hematoma, pseudoaneurysm, dissection, and arteriovenous fistula.[27] Contrast agents are generally nephrotoxic, although this risk can be reduced by the use of carbon dioxide angiography and preprocedure intravenous hydration.[25] However, carbon dioxide angiography may not be effective for visualization of more distal tibial and pedal vessels. As DSA can only effectively image endoluminal contrast, it also lacks the capability to characterize vessel wall and thrombus the way ultrasound and CTA can. As such, it can also underestimate plaque that is eccentric or has undergone outward remodeling.

THERAPEUTIC OPTIONS AND SURGICAL TECHNIQUES

Ultimately the treatment of PAD in diabetic patients can be broken down into 4 categories: nonoperative, amputation, surgical bypass, and endovascular intervention. General medical management of PAD in diabetic patients is outlined later in this article. In addition, it should be noted that nonoperative management should always be the first strategy applied in a patient presenting with claudication, and should also include a regular exercise regimen of repeatedly walking up to and into the level of claudicatory pain for at least 30 minutes per day, at least 4 days per week.

General Medical Management

It is important to recognize that although DM and peripheral vascular disease may have very concrete manifestations on the vasculature of extremities amenable to surgical intervention, they are systemic diseases requiring close medical management both in and out of the perioperative period. Both PAD and DM are coronary heart disease risk equivalents, meaning they have the same risk of cardiovascular events as patients with specifically coronary heart disease. This is especially important to consider when evaluating any patient for an operative intervention, as preoperative optimization is a necessity to reduce perioperative morbidity and mortality. The tenets of medical management are the controlling of glucose, blood pressure, and cholesterol, along with antiplatelet therapy.

Regarding glycemic control, ADA guidelines recommend a goal of less than 7.0% glycosylated hemoglobin (HbA1c). Hyperglycemia is a known to be a contributing risk factor to cardiovascular events; however, the degree of control necessary for protection has been much debated. More intensive glucose control has been studied in large trials, including Action to Control Cardiovascular Risk in Diabetes (ACCORD; intensive goal <6.0%), Action in Diabetes and Vascular Disease (ADVANCE; intensive goal <6.5%), and Veterans Affairs Diabetes Trial (VADT; intensive goal <6.0%). However, none of these studies showed reduction in cardiovascular events with more intense glucose control, and the ACCORD trial intensive control group had increased mortality from cardiovascular causes.[28–30]

Hypertension is already associated with a twofold to threefold increase in risk for claudication in PAD.[2] No studies, however, have directly linked hypertension with cardiovascular events in patients with PAD. In spite of this, other studies, including the United Kingdom Prospective Diabetes Study (UKPDS), showed diabetic end points and strokes have significantly reduced events when blood pressure is kept to a mean of 10 mm Hg lower.[31] Thus, current guidelines suggest a goal of 130/80 mm Hg. In the Heart Outcomes Prevention Evaluation (HOPE) trial, control of blood pressure by using an angiotensin-converting enzyme (ACE) inhibitor, ramipril, showed significantly reduced death, stroke, and myocardial infarction.[32] No specific prospective trials exist for patients with PAD and DM, but given these encouraging results, the 130/80 mm Hg blood pressure goal with ACE-inhibitor therapy, while appropriate, is supported by consensus.

Likewise, no specific trials exist looking at patients with PAD for cholesterol-lowering therapy but several large studies with large PAD subgroups support certain cholesterol goals. The Scandinavian Simvastatin Survival Study noted reduction in cholesterol levels reduced the risk of new or progressive claudication.[33] The Collaborative Atorvastatin Diabetes Study (CARDS) examined statins in patients solely with type 2 DM, and demonstrated a significant reduction in cardiovascular events irrespective of baseline low-density lipoprotein (LDL) level.[34] These data have ultimately led the ADA to recommend goal LDL levels of less than 100 mg/dL in patients with either cardiovascular disease or DM and less than 70 mg/dL in patients with both.[35]

Considering antiplatelet therapy, aspirin is already recommended as standard for patients with DM, although evidence for its benefits in PAD alone remain equivocal.[36] In contrast, the Clopidogrel versus Aspirin in Patients at Risk of Ischemic Events (CAPRIE) study, evaluating the 2 drugs in 19,000 patients, had a 6000-patient PAD subgroup showing a 24% risk reduction in myocardial infarction, stroke, and vascular death for clopidogrel over aspirin.[37] Thus, there is level B evidence for clopidogrel in patients with PAD and DM.

In summary, patients with DM and PAD should receive optimal medical management with goal HbA1c less than 7.0%, blood pressure lower than 130/80, LDL lower than 70 mg/dL, and antiplatelet therapy with at least aspirin and possibly clopidogrel.

Open Surgical Options

Indications for surgical and endovascular intervention include severe lifestyle-limiting claudication, pain while at rest, and nonhealing ulcers. This history should be taken in the context of the other diagnostic information acquired in the workup outlined previously. Other inclusion criteria for intervention include a viable limb postintervention that will contribute to the patient's quality of life. Bedridden and nonambulatory patients, or those who have sustained complications after repeated interventions, may be better candidates for further nonoperative management or amputation. This should be discussed with the patient/caregivers and reflect their goals as well.

If revascularization is to be pursued, the long-held gold standard intervention is an arterial bypass graft with autologous saphenous vein graft with establishment of straight-line pulsatile flow to a target ulcer if present. A 20-year review of lower extremity revascularization studies reaffirmed this position that the saphenous vein has the best results in all positions over time regardless of inflow or outflow vessel.[38] Femoropoliteal bypass, the most common bypass procedure, showed 5-year and 10-year patency rates of 83% and 63%, respectively, with a limb salvage rates of 89%.

Due to the increasing availability of surgery, repeat revascularization surgery, and other surgery, such as coronary artery bypass grafting; saphenous vein is often not an option for revascularization conduit. In this case, polytetrafluoroethylene grafts have become increasingly common as bypass conduits, although they have lower patency compared with autologous vein. Reported 5-year and 10-year patency rates in the same review were 62% and 24%, with limb salvage rates of 71% and 68%.[38] It should be noted for both open surgical and endovascular revascularization that limb salvage rates are usually greater than patency rates of the bypass conduit or treated vessel. A temporary increase in blood flow and oxygenation to a lesion may be enough to support ulcer healing and salvage a limb before the conduit occludes, so it is important to examine these meaningful outcomes when considering revascularization strategies.

Diabetic patients with PAD tend to have more infrapopliteal disease. For these patients, the femoropopliteal bypass grafts already mentioned may be important in reestablishing a high-pressure inflow vessel; however, more distal revascularization is often necessary. For these patients, pedal bypass grafts may be needed. There are few high-quality studies on these types of grafts. One review notes 10 studies reporting the results of pedal bypass grafting with median limb salvages rates at 1, 3, and 5 years of 86.0%, 88.5%, and 78.0%, respectively.[39]

With regard to these distal revascularizations, an emerging concept is that of angiosomes: an anatomic unit of tissue fed predominantly by one source artery. Six angiosomes are described for the foot[40]:

- Posterior tibial artery (3): calcaneal branch (heel), medial plantar artery (instep), lateral plantar artery (lateral midfoot and forefoot)
- Peroneal artery (2): anterior perforating branch (lateral anterior upper ankle), calcaneal branch (plantar heel)
- Anterior tibial artery (1): dorsalis pedis artery (dorsum of foot)

One retrospective analysis of 52 surgical bypasses examined a group of patients having direct revascularization of an ischemic angiosome versus another group with indirect revascularization. The direct revascularization group had a wound-healing rate of 91% versus a 62% rate in the indirect group.[41] Although this is only a small retrospective study, further examination of this concept may lead to new revascularization strategies in the future.

It should be noted that there are no major studies, including a matched control group, for noninterventional therapy. Data are available on the outcomes of patients with DM and critical limb ischemia (CLI) who were not revascularized, demonstrating a 1-year limb salvage rate of 54%.[42] This would seem to be lower than the often reported rates of approximately 70% to 90% in most revascularizations, although publication bias should be considered. Another study of patients with PAD and foot ulcers, 70% of whom had DM, examined treatment without revascularization. It reported a 1-year amputation rate of 23%, although 52% had complete wound closure in the same amount of time.[43]

Endovascular Options

Endovascular treatment of PAD is a rapidly evolving field with many new techniques and devices still under testing and study. Surgical bypass is generally the more durable revascularization option when possible; however, the indications for endovascular treatment are essentially the same as surgical bypass. An endovascular approach may also be preferable for patients at high risk for surgery, those without adequate autologous vein for bypass, and those with poor targets for surgical anastomoses or poor outflow vessels. In many centers, endovascular therapy is also now becoming the first-line option for revascularization.

Endovascular interventions are performed typically under local anesthesia, with direct puncture of the common femoral artery. Antegrade puncture may be made in the common femoral artery of the limb at risk. Once angiography of the affected vessels is performed, the intervention plan can be made. Many new emerging techniques and devices are available for intervention on identified lesions; however, balloon angioplasty is the simplest and most studied. It should be the first intervention performed.

Similar to surgical bypass, straight-line pulsatile flow to the foot is the ultimate goal of endovascular intervention. Anatomic outflow arteries are preferable targets, although large collateral vessels may also be intervened on. A large retrospective analysis of 1268 patients with CLI undergoing infrapopliteal percutaneous transluminal angioplasty (PTA) showed that the number of patent vessels is the most important predictor of limb salvage rates after infrapopliteal PTA; 1-year salvage rates for 0, 1, 2, and 3 patent infrapopliteal arteries were 56.4%, 73.1%, 80.4%, and 83.0% respectively.[44] The more patent vessels postintervention, the more likely limb salvage will be. The previously mentioned concept of angiosomes seems to hold true for PTA as well. Single-center retrospective data have shown improved results for direct revascularization of affected angiosomes.[45]

It is remains as yet difficult to compare outcomes between open surgical bypass and PTA for diabetic patients and infrapopliteal disease. The large, multicenter, randomized UK Bypass versus Angioplasty in Severe Ischemia of the Leg (BASIL) trial compared 452 patients with femoropopliteal disease and severe limb ischemia. It showed no significant differences in amputation-free survival, all-cause mortality, or quality of life between surgical and PTA groups. The angioplasty group did have a significantly higher reintervention rate of 28% compared with 17% for the surgical group.[46] However, only 42% of patients were diabetic and only one-third of the bypass group had a crural artery graft.

One study compared a series of patients (262 who underwent endovascular intervention, and 761 surgical revascularizations) with crural or pedal interventions. Five-year leg salvage rates were similar, 75.3% versus 76%, as were amputation-free survival rates, 37.3% versus 37.3%.[47] However, this was not a prospective, randomized trial.

Another concern in relation to endovascular intervention is the method of recanalization of occluded arteries. Transluminal should be the first option taken if possible. Another option in the crural vessels is subintimal recanalization. This procedure involves creating a dissection in the subintimal plane to cross an occluded segment of the vessel and then reenter the true arterial lumen distal to the lesion. The dissection plane can then be expanded using an angioplasty balloon to, in effect, create a bypass of the original occluded vessel lumen. Balloon inflation time may need to be prolonged up to 2 minutes sometimes; however, patency rates have been shown to be acceptable. Meta-analysis of this technique shows a primary patency of 55.8% at 12 months, with associated limb salvage rates of 80% to 90%. However, at 4 years, limb salvage decreases to as low as 34%.[48,49] Both transluminal and subintimal routes can be retreated again as needed.

A variety of new devices and techniques are also emerging in the endovascular field. Drug-eluting balloons, bare metal stents, drug-eluting stents, bioabsorbable stents, mechanical atherectomy, laser atherectomy, and cryoplasty are all available now. Although some will certainly offer effective treatment modalities in the future, these devices are beyond the scope of discussion for this article and currently do not have adequate evidence to clearly support their use in diabetic patients with PAD.

When performing endovascular interventions, it is essential for vascular interventionalists to consider the long-term consequences of any treatment modality beyond the thought of patency rates and the healing of a single ulcer. As yet, surgical bypass remains the most durable and effective revascularization option for patients. The risks and benefits of any endovascular intervention that would compromise a future surgical bypass, such as stenting of a possible future anastomotic site, must be weighed heavily before being performed.

SUMMARY

PAD and DM are both rapidly increasing in prevalence throughout the world. One may frequently coexist with the other and impose enormous health care costs on society, especially during their late phase of disease progression to lower extremity ischemia. It is important to be able to understand and diagnose each entity alone and together, as their coexistence can have direct implications for subsequent workup and intervention. CTA is the new standard in imaging for PAD for both diagnostic and interventional planning purposes. Patients should first be treated nonoperatively and with appropriate medical management with regard to blood sugar, blood pressure, cholesterol, and antiplatelet therapy; however, many will still ultimately need some form of revascularization to restore straight-line pulsatile flow to the foot. Open surgical bypass is generally thought to be the most durable and effective option in vascular surgery; however, no high-quality studies have compared surgery to endovascular therapy in diabetic patients with PAD and infrapopliteal disease. PTA is the first and most reliable endovascular intervention, although many new therapies are emerging. Further study and comparison of surgical bypass, PTA, and newer endovascular therapies is warranted and offers new promise for future treatments.

REFERENCES

1. Pearson WS. Ten-year comparison of estimates of overweight and obesity, diagnosed diabetes and use of office-based physician services for treatment of diabetes in the United States. Prev Med 2007;45:353–7.
2. Cronenwett JL, Johnston KW, Rutherford RB, et al. Rutherford's vascular surgery. 7th edition. Philadelphia: Saunders/Elsevier; 2010.
3. Criqui MH, Langer RD, Fronek A, et al. Mortality over a period of 10 years in patients with peripheral arterial disease. N Engl J Med 1992;326:381–6.
4. Hiatt WR, Hoag S, Hamman RF. Effect of diagnostic criteria on the prevalence of peripheral arterial disease. The San Luis Valley Diabetes Study. Circulation 1995; 91:1472–9.
5. Peach G, Griffin M, Jones KG, et al. Diagnosis and management of peripheral arterial disease. BMJ 2012;345:e5208.
6. Norgren L, Hiatt WR, Dormandy JA, et al. Inter-society consensus for the management of peripheral arterial disease (TASC II). J Vasc Surg 2007;45(Suppl S):S5–67.
7. Selvin E, Marinopoulos S, Berkenblit G, et al. Meta-analysis: glycosylated hemoglobin and cardiovascular disease in diabetes mellitus. Ann Intern Med 2004; 141:421–31.
8. Effect of intensive diabetes management on macrovascular events and risk factors in the Diabetes Control and Complications Trial. Am J Cardiol 1995;75: 894–903.
9. Eisenbarth GS. Type I diabetes mellitus. A chronic autoimmune disease. N Engl J Med 1986;314:1360–8.
10. DeFronzo RA. Lilly lecture 1987. The triumvirate: beta-cell, muscle, liver. A collusion responsible for NIDDM. Diabetes 1988;37:667–87.
11. Beckman JA, Creager MA, Libby P. Diabetes and atherosclerosis: epidemiology, pathophysiology, and management. JAMA 2002;287:2570–81.
12. Montagnani M, Golovchenko I, Kim I, et al. Inhibition of phosphatidylinositol 3-kinase enhances mitogenic actions of insulin in endothelial cells. J Biol Chem 2002; 277:1794–9.
13. Libby P. Inflammation in atherosclerosis. Nature 2002;420:868–74.
14. American Diabetes Association. Diagnosis and classification of diabetes mellitus. Diabetes Care 2011;34(Suppl 1):S62–9.
15. Jude EB, Oyibo SO, Chalmers N, et al. Peripheral arterial disease in diabetic and nondiabetic patients: a comparison of severity and outcome. Diabetes Care 2001;24:1433–7.
16. De Vivo S, Palmer-Kazen U, Kalin B, et al. Risk factors for poor collateral development in claudication. Vasc Endovascular Surg 2005;39:519–24.
17. McDaniel MD, Cronenwett JL. Basic data related to the natural history of intermittent claudication. Ann Vasc Surg 1989;3:273–7.

18. Edmonds ME, Morrison N, Laws JW, et al. Medial arterial calcification and diabetic neuropathy. Br Med J (Clin Res Ed) 1982;284:928–30.

19. Boyko EJ, Ahroni JH, Davignon D, et al. Diagnostic utility of the history and physical examination for peripheral vascular disease among patients with diabetes mellitus. J Clin Epidemiol 1997;50:659–68.

20. Lozano RM, Fernandez ML, Hernandez DM, et al. Validating the probe-to-bone test and other tests for diagnosing chronic osteomyelitis in the diabetic foot. Diabetes Care 2010;33:2140–5.

21. Schaper NC, Andros G, Apelqvist J, et al. Diagnosis and treatment of peripheral arterial disease in diabetic patients with a foot ulcer. A progress report of the International Working Group on the Diabetic Foot. Diabetes Metab Res Rev 2012; 28:218–24.

22. Tang GL, Chin J, Kibbe MR. Advances in diagnostic imaging for peripheral arterial disease. Expert Rev Cardiovasc Ther 2010;8:1447–55.

23. Moneta GL, Yeager RA, Lee RW, et al. Noninvasive localization of arterial occlusive disease: a comparison of segmental Doppler pressures and arterial duplex mapping. J Vasc Surg 1993;17:578–82.

24. Bandyk DF. Surveillance after lower extremity arterial bypass. Perspect Vasc Surg Endovasc Ther 2007;19:376–83 [discussion: 84–5].

25. Heijenbrok-Kal MH, Kock MC, Hunink MG. Lower extremity arterial disease: multidetector CT angiography meta-analysis. Radiology 2007;245:433–9.

26. Met R, Bipat S, Legemate DA, et al. Diagnostic performance of computed tomography angiography in peripheral arterial disease: a systematic review and meta-analysis. JAMA 2009;301:415–24.

27. Koelemay MJ, Lijmer JG, Stoker J, et al. Magnetic resonance angiography for the evaluation of lower extremity arterial disease: a meta-analysis. JAMA 2001;285: 1338–45.

28. Abraira C, Duckworth WC, Moritz T. Glycaemic separation and risk factor control in the Veterans Affairs Diabetes Trial: an interim report. Diabetes Obes Metab 2009;11:150–6.

29. Gerstein HC, Miller ME, Byington RP, et al. Effects of intensive glucose lowering in type 2 diabetes. N Engl J Med 2008;358:2545–59.

30. Patel A, MacMahon S, Chalmers J, et al. Intensive blood glucose control and vascular outcomes in patients with type 2 diabetes. N Engl J Med 2008;358: 2560–72.

31. Tight blood pressure control and risk of macrovascular and microvascular complications in type 2 diabetes: UKPDS 38. UK Prospective Diabetes Study Group. BMJ 1998;317:703–13.

32. Yusuf S, Sleight P, Pogue J, et al. Effects of an angiotensin-converting-enzyme inhibitor, ramipril, on cardiovascular events in high-risk patients. The Heart Outcomes Prevention Evaluation Study Investigators. N Engl J Med 2000;342:145–53.

33. Kjekshus J, Pedersen TR. Reducing the risk of coronary events: evidence from the Scandinavian Simvastatin Survival Study (4S). Am J Cardiol 1995;76:64C–8C.

34. Colhoun HM, Betteridge DJ, Durrington PN, et al. Primary prevention of cardiovascular disease with atorvastatin in type 2 diabetes in the Collaborative Atorvastatin Diabetes Study (CARDS): multicentre randomised placebo-controlled trial. Lancet 2004;364:685–96.

35. Brunzell JD, Davidson M, Furberg CD, et al. Lipoprotein management in patients with cardiometabolic risk: consensus conference report from the American Diabetes Association and the American College of Cardiology Foundation. J Am Coll Cardiol 2008;51:1512–24.

36. Colwell JA. Aspirin therapy in diabetes. Diabetes Care 2003;26(Suppl 1):S87–8.
37. CAPRIE Steering Committee. A randomised, blinded, trial of clopidogrel versus aspirin in patients at risk of ischaemic events (CAPRIE). CAPRIE Steering Committee. Lancet 1996;348:1329–39.
38. Ziegler KR, Muto A, Eghbalieh SD, et al. Basic data related to surgical infrainguinal revascularization procedures: a twenty year update. Ann Vasc Surg 2011;25: 413–22.
39. Hinchliffe RJ, Andros G, Apelqvist J, et al. A systematic review of the effectiveness of revascularization of the ulcerated foot in patients with diabetes and peripheral arterial disease. Diabetes Metab Res Rev 2012;28(Suppl 1):179–217.
40. Attinger CE, Evans KK, Bulan E, et al. Angiosomes of the foot and ankle and clinical implications for limb salvage: reconstruction, incisions, and revascularization. Plast Reconstr Surg 2006;117:261S–93S.
41. Neville RF, Attinger CE, Bulan EJ, et al. Revascularization of a specific angiosome for limb salvage: does the target artery matter? Ann Vasc Surg 2009;23:367–73.
42. Lepantalo M, Matzke S. Outcome of unreconstructed chronic critical leg ischaemia. Eur J Vasc Endovasc Surg 1996;11:153–7.
43. Marston WA, Davies SW, Armstrong B, et al. Natural history of limbs with arterial insufficiency and chronic ulceration treated without revascularization. J Vasc Surg 2006;44:108–14.
44. Peregrin JH, Koznar B, Kovac J, et al. PTA of infrapopliteal arteries: long-term clinical follow-up and analysis of factors influencing clinical outcome. Cardiovasc Intervent Radiol 2010;33:720–5.
45. Alexandrescu V, Vincent G, Azdad K, et al. A reliable approach to diabetic neuro-ischemic foot wounds: below-the-knee angiosome-oriented angioplasty. J Endovasc Ther 2011;18:376–87.
46. Adam DJ, Beard JD, Cleveland T, et al. Bypass versus angioplasty in severe ischaemia of the leg (BASIL): multicentre, randomised controlled trial. Lancet 2005;366:1925–34.
47. Soderstrom MI, Arvela EM, Korhonen M, et al. Infrapopliteal percutaneous transluminal angioplasty versus bypass surgery as first-line strategies in critical leg ischemia: a propensity score analysis. Ann Surg 2010;252:765–73.
48. Bown MJ, Bolia A, Sutton AJ. Subintimal angioplasty: meta-analytical evidence of clinical utility. Eur J Vasc Endovasc Surg 2009;38:323–37.
49. Met R, Van Lienden KP, Koelemay MJ, et al. Subintimal angioplasty for peripheral arterial occlusive disease: a systematic review. Cardiovasc Intervent Radiol 2008; 31:687–97.

New Modalities in the Chronic Ischemic Diabetic Foot Management

Sherif Y. Shalaby, MD[a], Peter Blume, DPM, FACFAS[b],
Bauer E. Sumpio, MD, PhD, FACS[c],*

KEYWORDS

- Critical limb ischemia • Diabetic foot • Therapy • Future perspectives

KEY POINTS

- Stem cell therapy is safe and effective in chronic ischemic diabetic foot (CIDF) management, especially for patients without options for revascularization.
- Processed lipoaspirate cells autologous transplantation is a feasible new modality in CIDF with high patient tolerance.
- Lipo-prostaglandin E_1 (PGE_1) works by improvement of peripheral circulation in CIDF and provides a longer duration of action and fewer side effects.
- Granulocyte colony-stimulating factor (G-CSF) induces terminal differentiation and release and improves the function of neutrophils from the bone marrow. It can reduce the need for surgical interventions, especially amputations.
- Heberprot-P is a novel perilesional and intralesional injection drug that gives promising results when injected deep in the ulcer matrix of the CIFD.
- De Marco formula (DMF) is a combination of procaine hydrochloride and polyvinylpyrrolidone. It reduces the lesion area and contributes to a reduction of amputations rate in CIDF trials.
- Low-dose urokinase improves microvascular blood flow in the CIDF via decreasing plasma fibrinogen levels.
- Heparin-induced extracorporal low-density lipoprotein precipitation (HELP) directly removes fibrinogen levels from the cardiovascular system and improves microvascular circulation.

INTRODUCTION

Since the 1980s, the diabetic population has increased worldwide, with a tripling in the United States from 5.6 million to 20.9 million.[1] In 2006, there were 65,700

Disclosure Statement: None.
[a] Department of Vascular Surgery, Yale University School of Medicine, 310 Cedar Street, New Haven, CT 06510, USA; [b] Orthopedics and Rehabilitation, and Anesthesia, Yale University School of Medicine, New Haven, CT 06510, USA; [c] Department of Vascular Surgery, Department of Surgery, Yale University School of Medicine, 333 Cedar Street, New Haven, CT 06510, USA
* Corresponding author.
E-mail address: bauer.sumpio@yale.edu

Clin Podiatr Med Surg 31 (2014) 27–42
http://dx.doi.org/10.1016/j.cpm.2013.09.009
0891-8422/14/$ – see front matter © 2014 Elsevier Inc. All rights reserved.
podiatric.theclinics.com

nontraumatic lower limb amputations, of which more than 60% occurred in the diabetic population.[2] In general, the "rule of 15" is applicable in patients with diabetes: approximately 15% of all diabetic patients develop a foot or leg ulcer during their lifetime, 15% of ulcers develop osteomyelitis, and 15% of ulcers result in amputation.[3] Lower limb amputations for diabetic ulceration contribute up to 85% of total cases.[4] The staggering number of nontraumatic lower limb amputations in the diabetic population emphasizes the vulnerability of their immunologic, wound healing, and tissue perfusion capacity to overcome the various external or internal factors causing ulcers.

The pathophysiology of diabetic ulceration is multifactorial and complex but the major underlying causes are peripheral neuropathy and ischemia from peripheral arterial disease (PAD).[5] The enigma of developing limb-threatening foot ulcers in patients with mild symptoms of arterial insufficiency occurs because the blood supply needed to allow healing of an ulcer, once one is present, is greater than that needed to maintain intact skin. The ulcer progresses to a chronic wound or gangrene unless the blood supply is improved.[6] PAD is common in the diabetic population because patients with diabetes ages 60 years or older are 2 to 3 times more likely to report an inability to walk one-quarter mile, climb stairs, or do housework compared with individuals without diabetes in the same age group.[2] Atherosclerosis has a higher incidence at a younger age in individuals with diabetes than in other individuals, and its hallmark is the involvement of the tibioperoneal vessels with sparing of the pedal vessels.[7] Neuropathy in patients with diabetes is usually distal symmetric sensorimotor polyneuropathy.[6] Emphasis should be placed on use of detection tools, such as the Semmes-Weinstein monofilament examination, which is a significant and independent predictor of future foot ulceration or likely future lower extremity amputations.[8] The diagnosis also comes at a substantial price to society, with a recent estimate of hospital costs for the care of a patient with critical limb ischemia (CLI) of $47,000.[9] According to the joint statement of the Society for Vascular Surgery and the American Podiatric Medical Association, interdisciplinary team cooperation exercises a pivotal role of reduction of time in management throughout the various diabetic foot conditions with salvage of the lower extremities as the ultimate goal.[10] New therapeutic modalities must be developed, however, when the interdisciplinary team approach is not sufficient to salvage the lower extremities in resistant diabetic ulcers.

Even though management of the ischemic diabetic foot has improved over the past decades with complex multidisciplinary teams, the advancement of modern vascular surgical reconstruction strategies, and improvements in endovascular techniques, the guidelines for management are vague other than the mainstays, such as early revascularization, appropriate prevention, infection control, and wound dressings. In general, the optimal strategy of CIDF management is to perform revascularization, if indicated, as soon as possible.[6]

The simultaneous high occurrence of PAD and foot ulcers in the diabetic population, however, has created a subset of patients with CIDF. This article discusses the efficiency, efficacy, and prognostic outcomes of the emerging new treatment modalities for the CIDF without options for revascularization (**Table 1**).

CELL THERAPY
Autologous Stem Cells Transplantation

Stem cell therapy is continuing to raise considerable interest in the field of PAD, specifically for CIDF, mainly due to the mild adverse effects and the lack of transplant

Table 1
Emerging therapeutic modalities for CIDF without options for revascularization

Cell Therapy	Drugs	Rheologic Treatment
Autologous stem cells	Prostaglandins	Lipid apheresis and rheopheresis
PLA cells	Low-dose urokinase	HELP
	G-CSF	
	Heberprot-P	
	DMF	

rejection because of autologous transplantation. The abundance and the availability of stem cells combined with techniques to successfully transplant stem cells to areas of lesion in the foot adds to the optimism. One drawback is that collecting stem cells from patients is a difficult and meticulous procedure and has become a critical research focus within treatment of CIDF patients. **Table 2** provides a summary of the new clinical trials of autologous stem cell transplantation for the CIDF. The two principal methods of administration of stem cells are by intra-arterial catheter antegrade with direct delivery to the distal artery of the affected limb or by multiple intramuscular injections. Both techniques have shown clinical improvement.[11,12] A majority of clinical trials, however, favor the use of the intramuscular route because it is difficult to deliver cells through diseased arteries in patients with limb ischemia. The intramuscular approach provides the most direct method of delivery of stem cells to the lesion of interest.

The exact dose and type of stem cells to be administered are not well defined.[13] Kirana and colleagues[14] demonstrated that use of only 40 mL of crude bone marrow aspirate yielded complete primary wound healing without any adverse effects. Further development of the various methods of autologous stem cell transplantation, such as reintervening by transplanting stem cells again for deteriorating patients, has been demonstrated in a clinical trial by Huang and colleagues,[15] with a 100% amputation rescue. It is the only clinical trial that reintervened for deteriorating patients on follow-up. The trial was not blinded, however, and had only a small size group of implanted stem cell patients (n = 14), emphasizing the need for larger blinded clinical trials. Moreover, the process of bone marrow aspiration for stem cell harvesting is associated with anemia and requires general anesthesia, which raises the question of whether acquisition of stem cells from bone marrow cells (BMCs) or peripheral blood progenitor cells (PBPCs) would differentially change the course of clinical outcome of patients. Dubsky and colleagues[16] reported no difference in clinical outcome between BMC and PBPC treatment, assessed by transcutaneous oxygen pressure (TcPO$_2$) measurements, because the arteries of patients with diabetes may be calcified.[6] Also, there was no evidence of systemic vasculogenesis between the two groups of stem cell lines–treated patients.

The exact beneficial mechanism of injected stem cells in ischemic tissues and the interaction between the cells and the matrix is unknown. The tissue matrix exerts its own effects on wound healing via complex interactions with regenerative cells. Extracellular matrix rigidity influences mesenchymal stem cell (MSC) fate decisions[17] and, based on progress in understanding biomechanical regulation of mesenchymal cell function, is leading to novel approaches for improving clinical outcomes in fibrotic diseases and wound healing.[18] Some investigators have combined endothelial cells with MSC to study vascular network formation in 3-D matrices.[19] They have demonstrated an inverse relationship between matrix stiffness and network formation. These findings suggest that tissue stiffness must be within a permissible range to promote

Table 2
Summary of current stem cell trials in CIDF patients

Trial	Patient State	Cell	Route	Dosage (No. of Cells/mL)	Inclusion Criteria	Exclusion Criteria	Outcome	Remarks
Kawamura et al,[52] 2005	CLI and DFU	PB-MNC	IM	$3.6 \pm 2.9 \times 10^7$ or $4.8 \pm 4.2 \times 10^7$	• RP • C • LU • Nonimproving symptoms with meds (PGE$_1$) ± anticoagulants	• NL • Active infection under poor control • MN • MI • ANPE • CVD	Blood flow↑ Ischemic limb rescue↑ 73% rescued from amputation	87.5% of amputations at $\leq 5 \times 10^7$ CD34
Huang et al,[15] 2005	CLI	PB-MNC	IM	3×10^9	DP with proved CLI	• HYCOA • GAGR above the ankle ± severe coronary, CVD, and RVD	Blood flow recovery ↑ New vessels formation ↑ 100% Amputation rescue (14/14) vs 64% (9/14) in control	Forty days after transplantation, the severely diseased lower limb was given an additional transplantation of the same number of the cells
Bartsch et al,[12] 2005	DFU	BM-MNC	IA + IM	157×10^6	—	—	Ulcer healing Walking distance ↑ Blood circulation ↑	One patient clinical trial
Vojtassak et al,[53] 2006	DFU	BMSC	TA	3×10^6	—	—	Ulcer healing	One patient clinical trial

Study		Cells	Route	Dose	Inclusion Criteria	Exclusion Criteria	Outcomes	Notes
Gabr et al,[54] 2011	CLI	BM-MNC	IM	1.11×10^9	• CLI (LU/GAGR) • No possible open surgical or endovascular interventional options	• RF • Dialysis • Active overwhelming infection in the affected limb that threatens the patient's life • PR, BMD	Limb perfusion↑ ABI↑ Amputation rescued 11/16 (69%)	50% of patients ≤ 60 y
Kirana et al,[25] 2012	DFU + CLI	BMC TRC	IM and IA	50×10^6 30×10^6	• DM 1 and 2 • 18–80 y old • DFU < Wagner stage III • CFU >6 wk • 1 wk of SWT • PAD stage III or IV (Fountaine classification) • CLI (ABI <0.7 ± TcPO$_2$ <30 mmHg) • No other therapeutic option	• Pregnancy • Psychological or mental disorder • HYCOA • Hx of AR • SHF (III–IV) • Therapy using vasoactive substance (prostaglandin) • HbA$_{1c}$ >8% • Hg <10 mg/dL • CICR <30 mL/min • DR • Systemic bacterial or viral infection (treponem, hepatitis, CMV, HIV, parvovirus B19, herpesvirus) • Sepsis • Previous stem cell and or growth factor therapy • Hx of malignancy less than 5 y before study start	Increased TcPO$_2$; 10/12 (83%) BMC + 8/10 (80%) TRC group amputation rescue	More than 80% of the patients presented with CHD and hypertension The average age was approximately 70 y

(continued on next page)

Table 2
(continued)

Trial	Patient State	Cell	Route	Dosage (No. of Cells/mL)	Inclusion Criteria	Exclusion Criteria	Outcome	Remarks
Dubsky et al,[16] 2013	DFU and CLI	BMSC + PB-MNC	IM	BMSC: 2.2 ± 1.5 × 10⁷ PBPC: 2.4 ± 2.2 × 10⁷	• DFD • CLI • RC (4–6) • Very severe angiographic finding not eligible for revascularization	• SLO • SHD • DVT (in past 6 mo) • PR • Known neoplasm	11.1% (Control) vs 50% amputation rate Increased TcPO₂	No difference between BMSC and PB-MNC No signs of systemic vasculogenesis

Abbreviations: AR, allergic reaction; ANPE, angina pectoris; BMC, bone marrow mononuclear cell; BMD, bone marrow disease; C, cyanosis; CFU, chronic foot ulcer; CHD, coronary heart disease; CICR, creatinine clearance; CMV, cytomegalovirus; CVD, cerebrovascular disease; DFD, diabetic foot disease; DFU, diabetic foot ulcer; DM, diabetes mellitus; DP, diabetic patients; DR, diabetic retinopathy; DVT, deep venous thrombosis; GAGR, gangrene; Hg, hemoglobin; Hx, History; HYCOA, hypercoaguablity; IA, intra-arterial; IM, intramuscular; LN, limb necrosis; LU, limb ulcer; MI, myocardial infarction; MN, malignant neoplasm; PAD, peripheral arterial disease; PB-MNC peripheral blood - mononuclear cells; PR, proliferative retinopathy severe hematological diseases; RC, Rutherford category; RF, Renal failure; RP, rest pain; RVD, renal vascular disease; SHD, severe hematological disease; SHF, severe heart failure; SLO, severe limb edema; SWT, standard wound treatment; TA, topical application; TRC, tissue repair cells are BMCs enriched in CD90+ cells.

vascularization, which has implications for angiogenesis in wound healing and fibrosis.[18] It makes biologic sense that the more fibrosis in the diabetic foot ulcer matrix, the more likely it hinders stem cells regenerative capabilities.

It is not clear whether stem cells are directly involved in angiogenesis or indirectly as cytokines factories with paracrine effects.[20] The most important of the angiogenic cytokines are vascular endothelial growth factors (VEGFs) and basic fibroblast growth factor (b-FGF), whose production are also regulated by other bioactive metabolic process, such as interferon gamma and interleukin-10.[21] Because the cytokines can disseminate and affect nontarget tissues, there is a potential side effect of proliferative retinopathy and stimulation of tumor growth.[22–24] It is also difficult to assess whether stem cell therapy could further complicate or reactivate tumors in CIDF patients due to the multiple patient trials that exclude cancer patients. None of the patients mentioned in the listed trials, however, died of cancer-related causes but rather of cardiovascular causes. The correlation of stem cell therapy and circulatory failure during therapy is also of great interest because VEGF is a potent growth and angiogenic cytokine.[16,25] Kajiguchi and colleagues[26] investigated angiogenic cytokines (VEGF, b-FGF, and angiopoietin-1) after stem cell therapy and found no difference in serum between responders and nonresponders to stem cell therapy. Moreover, most of the patients in this study were over 65 years old and presented with multiple comorbidities. Further studies that include the inclusion of cardiac and cancer patients with long-term follow-up are necessary to assess the overall cost effectiveness of stem therapy in this patient group.

The evolutionary course of stem cell clinical trials in CIDF patients has expanded not only the study groups receiving stem cells but also the different types of treated stem cells due to the solid evidence of their efficacy and safety. The focus of current investigations is on comparing different types of stem cell therapy clinical outcomes rather than simply stem cell therapy versus conventional therapy. For instance, Kirana and colleagues[25] examined the efficacy of tissue repair cells (TRCs), which are bone marrow–aspirated stem cells cultivated in a flow system. The single-pass perfusion enables fresh medium to flow slowly over cells without retention of waste metabolites or differentiating cytokines.[27] The trial proved the safety and feasibility of both TRC and BMC lines.

Finally, there is a strong optimism that stem cell therapy will become relevant in clinical practice, especially with the implementation of new beside centrifugation systems (eg, SmartPrep, Harvest Technologies, Plymouth, MA) that obviate complicated and skilled laboratory units. This progress will enable feasibility and wider access to CIDF patients in the future.[28]

Processed Lipoaspirate Cells

There is extensive research in using cell lines other than stem cells in the treatment of CIDF patients. Processed lipoaspirate (PLA) cells synergistically stimulate the activity of fibroblasts from patients with diabetes in vitro. The cells are collected by abdominal liposuction and then treated with collagenase type I and ammonium chloride (for red blood cell lysis). PLA cells are injected in the débrided wound after being suspended in fibrinogen and then sealed in the wound via thrombin application and Tegaderm.[29] PLA cells contain mast cells, pericytes, stem cells, endothelial cells, and fibroblasts, which are all postulated to hasten wound healing.

Fig. 1 shows the results of a clinical trial on PLA cells.[25] The inclusion criteria were diabetes mellitus type 1 and 2; resistant to healing for 6 weeks; Wagner score 1 and 2; T_cPO_2 greater than 30; and ankle-brachial index (ABI) greater than 0.5. Exclusion criteria were infection, cellulites, osteomyelitis (diagnosed by MRI and bacterial

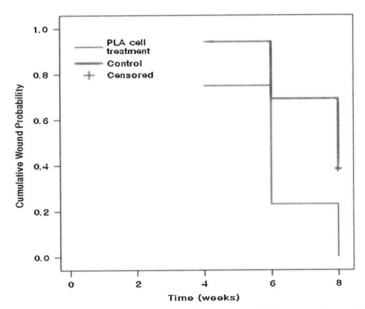

Fig. 1. Kaplan-Meier diagram showing the results on time of ulcer to reach complete healing (wound closure) by 8 weeks in PLA-treated group whereas only 62% complete healing in the control group. (*From* Han SK, Kim HR, Kim WK. The treatment of diabetic foot ulcers with uncultured, processed lipoaspirate cells: a pilot study. Wound Repair Regen 2010;18:342–8; with permission.)

culture results), chronic renal failure, hemoglobin A_{1c} (Hb A_{1c}) greater than 9%, no tolerance to offloading, and poor prognostic diseases. The control group was treated with only thrombin and fibrinogen. The patients returned every 3 to 7 days for wound examination and dressing change. The injection dosage was $4.0–8.0 \times 10^6$ cells/mL. Two patients were excluded after developing an overt clinical infection and the remaining 26 patients were analyzed. All patients achieved wound healing after 8 weeks compared with 62% in the control group ($P<.05$) without adverse effects related to therapy. Complete healing ranged from 17 to 56 days (mean, 33.8 ± 11.6 days) in the PLA cell–treated group and from 28 to 56 days (mean, 42.1 ± 9.5 days) in the control group ($P<.05$).

Table 3 summarizes overall benefits and limitations of the clinical trial. PLA cells can offer a good prognostic outcome for difficult-to-treat diabetic foot patients. Large double-blind trials are needed, however, before initiation into widespread clinical practice.

Table 3	
Overall benefits and limitations of LPA therapy clinical trial	
Benefits	**Limitations**
No associated bone marrow aspiration or cryoprecipitate complications	Collagenase has adverse effects on wounds
PLA cells easy to obtain in large quantities	Low yield of cell aspirated in elderly compared with healthy
Minimal adverse effects	Study is nonblinded
Excellent healing rates	May require multiple operating room procedures

DRUGS
Prostaglandins

Prostaglandins are not a new modality for treatment of CLI but trials determining their efficacy and safety for CIDF are scarce. The most common prostaglandin used is PGE_1, which improves the peripheral circulation via its platelet inhibitory action and vasodilatory effects. Their mechanisms are thought to play a role in enhancement of neovascularization of granulation tissue.

Lipo-PGE_1 is PGE_1 incorporated into lipid microspheres, which prevents inactivation by the lungs, provides a longer duration of action, and causes fewer side effects. The drug is superior to conventional PGE_1 due to its ability to accumulate in inflammatory lesions and blood vessels due its lipid microsphere distribution.[30] It is widely used as a nutrient infusion in standard clinical practice. A large clinical trial[31] investigated lipo-PGE_1 injection in 409 patients in 108 Japanese medical institutions from June 2004 to July 2007. The study was a prospective observational study that included ischemic, neuropathic, and neuroischemic diabetic foot ulcers with nonacute infection that did not require surgical debridement during the survey period. It excluded those who had contraindications to the drug, severe heart failure, hemorrhage, known or suspected pregnancy, and hypersensitivity to the drug or its components. In the trial, the dose administered was 5 µg to 10 µg of the drug once daily for 4 weeks. As a comparison, the dose of conventional PGE_1 is 40 µg twice a day over 2 to 4 hours intraarterially or intravenously.[32] The incidence of adverse effects, consisting of gastric hemorrhage, pleural effusion, and congestive heart failure, was 4.1%. Overall ulcer size reduction rate in the study was 42.5% ± 3.4%. The reduction by ulcer type was 34.0% for ischemic, 61.8% for neuropathic, and 33% for neuroischemic ulcers (**Fig. 2**). The treatment was significantly more effective for neuropathic than for ischemic ulcers. The limitation of the trial was that it was a postmarketing survey using current standard diagnostic criteria, there were no restrictions to preexisting therapeutic regimens, and it indicated neither the prevalence of foot amputations nor complete

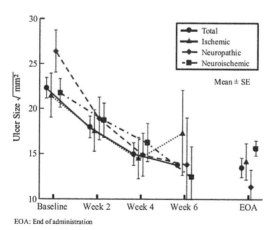

Fig. 2. Miyata and colleagues'[31] trial comparing ulcer size reduction in patients treated with lipo-PGE_1. Ulcer size at onset of administration was largest for neuropathic ulcer and was reduced in all ulcer types but neuropathic ulcer was the smallest at the end of administration. (*From* Miyata T, Yamada N, Miyachi Y. Efficacy by ulcer type and safety of lipo-PGE1 for Japanese patients with diabetic foot ulcers. J Atheroscler Thromb 2010;17:805–16; with permission.)

wound healing. Nevertheless, there was overall improvement in patients who were not excluded due to their foot infection and necrotic lesions.

The Inter-Society Consensus for the Management of Peripheral Arterial Disease (TASC II) does not recommend PGE_1[33] whereas the German Society of Angiology and Vascular Surgery supports it with level of evidence A. This latter conclusion was based, however, on older studies and in agreement with the prior experiences of the authors of this guideline.[34] Furthermore, larger double-blind clinical trials are recommended to justify the implementation of lipo-PGE_1 in wide clinical practice and formulation of guidelines specific to CIDF because none exists.

Granulocyte Colony-Stimulating Factor

G-CSF is an endogenous hematopoietic growth factor that induces terminal differentiation and release of neutrophils from the bone marrow. G-CSF stimulates the growth and improves the function of both normal and defective neutrophils.[35] It is hypothesized to improve the defective neutrophils of diabetic patients and those who have diabetic foot ulcers.[36]

A recent meta-analysis of the utility of G-CSF[37] included 5 studies that enrolled 167 patients and randomized 85 to receive G-CSF and 82 to control. Using G-CSF was associated with a significantly reduced likelihood of lower extremity surgical intervention (relative risk [RR] 0.37; 95% CI, 0.20–0.68), amputation (RR 0.41; 95% CI, 0.18–0.95), and hospital stay (mean difference 1.40 days; 95% CI, −2.27 to −0.53 days.) A low number needed to treat (NNT) has been demonstrated for overall surgical interventions (NNT = 5) and for amputation (NNT = 9), suggesting that G-CSF is an appropriate intervention in patients with limb-threatening infections.[37] Regarding drug safety, only 10 patients in 1 study reported adverse effects, such as increased serum alkaline phosphatase, transit bone pain, and skin efflorescence. The investigators concluded, "G-CSF is expensive and given the lack of evidence that G-CSF therapy can help cure infections or heal ulcers, one might conclude there is little reason to use it, especially for mild infections. If, on the other hand, it can reduce the need for surgical interventions, especially amputations, it may be worth providing where possible."

Heberprot-P

Heberprot-P is a novel Cuban drug containing recombinant human epidermal growth factor (EGF) for perilesional and intralesional infiltration.[38] Administration of EGF on wounds is not a new modality but when applied topically to wounds to promote tissue healing it had poor initial results.[39] The site of Heberprot-P injection is crucial to its efficacy due to the contemporary evidence that EGF injected into the ulcer matrix may result in an association complex with extracellular matrix proteins, thus enhancing cell proliferation and migration.[40] Superficial administration of Heberprot-P decreases its efficacy due to the occupancy of fibroblasts populating the more superficial stratum expressing more prohibitin and far fewer EGF receptors.[38] Prohibitin is a known inhibitor of cell cycle progression.[41]

EGF infiltration in poor-prognosis wounds increased and accelerated healing toward a rapid and sustained response. More than 80% granulation was obtained globally with Heberprot-P, in comparison with less than 60% with standard care alone. Of patients treated with Heberprot-P (75 µg 3 times per week until complete granulation or for a maximum of 8 weeks) in association with standard care, 77% healed; only 56% healed with placebo injections and standard care.[42] The most frequent adverse events were tremors, chills, pain, and an intense burning sensation at site of administration and local infection.[43] Heberprot-P has potential on the world market; it is approved in 15 countries (mainly South America) as an adjuvant therapy for diabetic foot ulcers.

De Marco Formula

DMF is a combination of procaine hydrochloride and polyvinylpyrrolidone (a synthetic hydrophilizing polymer that accumulates in the skin). Procaine induces reduction of free radical generation, vasodilation, and lysosomal enzyme release from rabbit and human polymorphonuclear leukocyte that could contribute to lesion area tissue damage prevention.

An uncontrolled study done in Cuba,[44] including 31 patients suffering from various diabetic foot problems, showed a 33% to 69% decrease in major amputation after treatment with conventional wound therapy plus intramuscular injections of DMF (0.15 mL/kg every 8 h; approximately 400 mg of procaine/dose) for 7 days. In another uncontrolled pilot study,[44] 34 patients who had an infected diabetic foot with history of 1 or more toe amputations or a surgical débridement with or without pervious procedures were treated with conventional wound therapy for diabetic foot plus DMF (0.15 mL/kg/d intramusacularly) for 10 days and then twice a week until healing of the lesions or completion of a 52-day period. Although, the trial resulted in 18% of patients (n = 6) requiring a lower limb amputation with the combined treatment, the standard reported rate in Cuba of major amputation is 25% to 29%. There was also a progressive reduction of the mean lesion area from 51.29 cm^2 at the end of the treatment was observed. A larger double-blind trial needs to assess whether DMF can be used as an adjuvant therapy to the diabetic foot.

RHEOLOGIC TREATMENT
Low-Dose Urokinase

Low-dose urkoinase has been used in the treatment of CIDF patients based on the widely accepted notion that fibrinogen is strongly, consistently, and independently related to cardiovascular risk. The evidence is based on prospective epidemiologic studies and clinical observations.[45] It is also known that fibrinogen tends to rise as an acute-phase protein in acutely infected diabetic foot syndrome. Fibrinogen is a crucial determinant of plasma viscosity and is partially responsible for a worsening of microvascular blood flow. A decrease in fibrinogen concentration combined with lysis of microthrombi in the microvasculature has been hypothesized as responsible for the effect of urokinase.[46] This results in improvement in microvascular blood flow of nutritive skin capillaries.

Weck and colleagues[47] conducted an open, prospective, noncontrolled, multicenter cohort study in 77 type 2 diabetic patients with CLI and diabetic foot ulceration. The trial included patients with angiopathic or angioneuropathic diabetic foot lesions, CLI, and no surgical or endovascular treatment option. A patient's plasma fibrinogen level had to exceed 4.0 g/L. The trial did not discuss exclusion of patients due to necrosis or infection of the foot ulcer. It mainly excluded patients with an increased risk of bleeding. During the trial, dosage was 1 IU if plasma fibrinogen greater than or equal to 2.5 g/L and 0.5 IU if fibrinogen less than 2.5 g/L. Treatment with urokinase was stopped if ulcer healing occurred before 21 doses had been administered and if plasma fibrinogen concentration dropped to less than 1.6 g/L. After 12 months, 33% of the surviving patients demonstrated completely healed ulcers, having no major amputation (**Fig. 3**). The total survival rate was 85%, amputation-free survival 69%, and rate of major amputation 21%. The adverse effects of urokinase are concerning, however, due to a 14.5% (n = 11) overall incidence with 3.9% (n = 3) incidence of

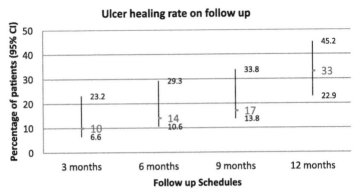

Fig. 3. Primary outcome of Weck and colleagues'[47] trial in 77 patients with type 2 diabetes mellitus—number of patients alive and having no major amputation and no further ischemic ulceration at 12 months' follow-up after short-term urokinase therapy. (*Adapted from* Weck M, Rietzsch H, Lawall H, et al. Intermittent intravenous urokinase for critical limb ischemia in diabetic foot ulceration. Thromb Haemost 2008;100(3):475–82; with permission.)

serious adverse effects, such as cerebral bleeding, transient hypotension, and bleeding into the lower limbs. The results of the trial are promising but bigger controlled, randomized, and double-blind studies need to be carried out before any serious consideration of incorporating urokinase into a wider clinical practice.

Heparin-Induced Extracorporal Low-Density Lipoprotein Precipitation in Diabetic Foot Syndrome

On the same principle of lowering fibrinogen levels in the blood using urokinase, HELP apheresis is a direct rapid intervention on fibrinogen via its removal from the circulation by vascular access, often requiring an arteriovenous fistula.[48] HELP apheresis lowers lipid fractions, providing acute improvement of whole blood and plasma viscosity and thus optimizing the microcirculation.[49]

In a clinical trial by Rietzsch and colleagues,[50] 17 diabetic patients with septic foot lesions were enrolled. Inclusion criteria were patients noneligible for revascularization due to severe angiopathy, systemic infection (leukocytosis or lymphadenitis), high risk for amputation, and plasma fibrinogen greater than 6 g/L. Exclusion criteria were patients with an indication for revascularization or thrombectomy, known hemorrhagic diathesis, gastrointestinal ulcers, cancer, liver disease, apoplexy, or cardiac insufficiency. All patients underwent HELP apheresis regularly to remove low-density lipoproteins, fibrinogen, and lipoprotein from plasma until fibrinogen levels were stabilized at 3 g/L or infection was controllable as evidenced by alleviation of necrosis. Mean fibrinogen levels dropped to 2.76 (0.36–5.30) after HELP apheresis treatment. The outcome, an only 18% amputation rate (**Fig. 4**), would be considered stellar considering the comorbidities and presenting conditions of the patients in the trial. The intensive patient health care duration, however, was on average 111 days and all the patients were closely monitored for control of blood sugars. Also, the trial had no control group nor was it blinded. The results of the trial encourage creating larger controlled and blinded trials with patients having different statuses of overall health to accurately assess HELP apheresis effectiveness for patients who fail conventional therapy.

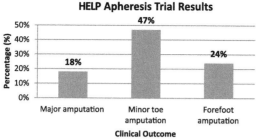

Fig. 4. HELP apheresis clinical trial outcome of 17 patients with diabetes, associated comorbidities, and challenging presenting conditions. (*From* Rietzsch H, Panzner I, Selisko T, et al. Heparin-induced Extracorporal LDL precipitation (H.E.L.P) in diabetic foot syndrome - preventive and regenerative potential? Horm Metab Res 2008;40(7):487–90; with permission.)

SUMMARY

As patient populations with diabetes and CIDF ulcers increase, new treatment options will also increase, which will further invigorate the need of management guidelines because optimal management can reduce the number of amputations, prevent infection, decrease the probability of ulceration, maintain skin integrity, and improve function for patients with foot ulcers.[6] The guidelines to be constructed under a wide consensus, which ultimately result in increasing quality and decreasing costs of health care to patients. Aside from health care providers, patient education is essential for reduction of risk factors and for early recognition of foot complications.[51] Although the results of new modalities in the CIDF management are promising in the context of a multitude of clinical trials of rigorous standardization via various definitions and methods, further analysis is required before the inclusion of this aforementioned modality into a standard clinical practice.

REFERENCES

1. Available at: www.cdc.gov/diabetes/statistics/prev/national/figpersons.htm. Accessed April, 2013.
2. Available at: www.cdc.gov/diabetes/pubs/estimates11.htm#12. Accessed April, 2013.
3. Ramsey SD, Newton K, Blough D, et al. Incidence, outcomes, and cost of foot ulcers in patients with diabetes. Diabetes Care 1999;22(3):382–7.
4. Reiber GE, Vileikyte L, Boyko EJ, et al. Causal pathways for incident lower-extremity ulcers in patients with diabetes from two settings. Diabetes Care 1999;22(1):157–62.
5. Bowering CK. Diabetic foot ulcers. Pathophysiology, assessment, and therapy. Can Fam Physician 2001;47:1007–16.
6. Sumpio BE. Foot ulcers. N Engl J Med 2000;343(11):787–93.
7. Kamal K, Powell RJ, Sumpio BE. The pathobiology of diabetes mellitus: implications for surgeons. J Am Coll Surg 1996;183(3):271–89.
8. Feng Y, Schlosser FJ, Sumpio BE. The Semmes Weinstein monofilament examination is a significant predictor of the risk of foot ulceration and amputation in patients with diabetes mellitus. J Vasc Surg 2011;53(1):220–6.e1–5.
9. Rajagopalan S, Dean SM, Mohler ER III, et al, editors. Manual of Vascular Diseases. Second Edition. Philadelphia: Wolters Kluwer, Lippincott Williams & Wilkins; 2012. p. 626.

10. Sumpio BE, Armstrong DG, Lavery LA, et al, SVS/APMA Writing Group. The role of interdisciplinary team approach in the management of the diabetic foot: a joint statement from the Society for Vascular Surgery and the American Podiatric Medical Association. J Vasc Surg 2010;51(6):1504–6.

11. Tateishi-Yuyama E, Matsubara H, Murohara T, et al. Therapeutic angiogenesis for patients with limb ischaemia by autologous transplantation of bone-marrow cells: a pilot study and a randomised controlled trial. Lancet 2002;360(9331): 427–35.

12. Bartsch T, Brehm M, Falke T, et al. Rapid healing of a therapy-refractory diabetic foot after transplantation of autologous bone marrow stem cells. [Schnelle Abheilung eines therapierefraktaren diabetischen Fusses nach autologer Knochenmarkstammzelltransplantation]. Med Klin 2005;100(10):676–80 [in German].

13. Lawall H, Bramlage P, Amann B. Stem cell and progenitor cell therapy in peripheral artery disease. A critical appraisal. Thromb Haemost 2010;103(4): 696–709.

14. Kirana S, Stratmann B, Lammers D, et al. Wound therapy with autologous bone marrow stem cells in diabetic patients with ischaemia-induced tissue ulcers affecting the lower limbs. Int J Clin Pract 2007;61(4):690–2.

15. Huang P, Li S, Han M, et al. Autologous transplantation of granulocyte colony-stimulating factor-mobilized peripheral blood mononuclear cells improves critical limb ischemia in diabetes. Diabetes Care 2005;28(9):2155–60.

16. Dubsky M, Jirkovska A, Bem R, et al. Both autologous bone marrow mononuclear cells and peripheral blood progenitor cells therapies similarly improve ischemia in patients with diabetic foot in comparison with control treatment. Diabetes Metab Res Rev 2013;29(5):369–76.

17. Engler AJ, Sen S, Sweeney HL, et al. Matrix elasticity directs stem cell lineage specification. Cell 2006;126(4):677–89.

18. Tschumperlin DJ, Liu F, Tager AM. Biomechanical regulation of mesenchymal cell function. Curr Opin Rheumatol 2013;25(1):92–100.

19. Rao RR, Peterson AW, Ceccarelli J, et al. Matrix composition regulates three-dimensional network formation by endothelial cells and mesenchymal stem cells in collagen/fibrin materials. Angiogenesis 2012;15(2):253–64.

20. Aranguren XL, Verfaillie CM, Luttun A. Emerging hurdles in stem cell therapy for peripheral vascular disease. J Mol Med 2009;87(1):3–16.

21. Di Vita G, Patti R, D'Agostino P, et al. Serum VEGF and b-FGF profiles after tension-free or conventional hernioplasty. Langenbecks Arch Surg 2005;390(6): 528–33.

22. Amann B, Luedemann C, Ratei R, et al. Autologous bone marrow cell transplantation increases leg perfusion and reduces amputations in patients with advanced critical limb ischemia due to peripheral artery disease. Cell Transplant 2009;18(3):371–80.

23. Matoba S, Tatsumi T, Murohara T, et al. Long-term clinical outcome after intramuscular implantation of bone marrow mononuclear cells (Therapeutic Angiogenesis by Cell Transplantation [TACT] trial) in patients with chronic limb ischemia. Am Heart J 2008;156(5):1010–8.

24. Miyamoto K, Nishigami K, Nagaya N, et al. Unblinded pilot study of autologous transplantation of bone marrow mononuclear cells in patients with thromboangiitis obliterans. Circulation 2006;114(24):2679–84.

25. Kirana S, Stratmann B, Prante C, et al. Autologous stem cell therapy in the treatment of limb ischaemia induced chronic tissue ulcers of diabetic foot patients. Int J Clin Pract 2012;66(4):384–93.

26. Kajiguchi M, Kondo T, Izawa H, et al. Safety and efficacy of autologous progenitor cell transplantation for therapeutic angiogenesis in patients with critical limb ischemia. Circ J 2007;71(2):196–201.
27. Rodriguez L, Azqueta C, Azzalin S, et al. Washing of cord blood grafts after thawing: high cell recovery using an automated and closed system. Vox Sang 2004;87(3):165–72.
28. Amann B, Ludemann C, Ruckert R, et al. Design and rationale of a randomized, double-blind, placebo-controlled phase III study for autologous bone marrow cell transplantation in critical limb ischemia: the BONe Marrow Outcomes Trial in Critical Limb Ischemia (BONMOT-CLI). Vasa 2008;37(4):319–25.
29. Han SK, Kim HR, Kim WK. The treatment of diabetic foot ulcers with uncultured, processed lipoaspirate cells: a pilot study. Wound Repair Regen 2010;18(4): 342–8.
30. Mizushima Y, Yanagawa A, Hoshi K. Prostaglandin E1 is more effective, when incorporated in lipid microspheres, for treatment of peripheral vascular diseases in man. J Pharm Pharmacol 1983;35(10):666–7.
31. Miyata T, Yamada N, Miyachi Y. Efficacy by ulcer type and safety of lipo-PGE1 for Japanese patients with diabetic foot ulcers. J Atheroscler Thromb 2010; 17(8):805–16.
32. Weck M, Slesaczeck T, Rietzsch H, et al. Noninvasive management of the diabetic foot with critical limb ischemia: current options and future perspectives. Ther Adv Endocrinol Metab 2011;2(6):247–55.
33. Norgren L, Hiatt WR, Dormandy JA, et al. Inter-society consensus for the management of peripheral arterial disease (TASC II). J Vasc Surg 2007;45(Suppl S): S5–67.
34. Lawall H, Gorriahn H, Amendt K, et al. Long-term outcomes after medical and interventional therapy of critical limb ischemia. Eur J Intern Med 2009;20(6): 616–21.
35. Nelson S, Heyder AM, Stone J, et al. A randomized controlled trial of filgrastim for the treatment of hospitalized patients with multilobar pneumonia. J Infect Dis 2000;182(3):970–3.
36. Sato N, Kashima K, Tanaka Y, et al. Effect of granulocyte-colony stimulating factor on generation of oxygen-derived free radicals and myeloperoxidase activity in neutrophils from poorly controlled NIDDM patients. Diabetes 1997;46(1): 133–7.
37. Cruciani M, Lipsky BA, Mengoli C, et al. Granulocyte-colony stimulating factors as adjunctive therapy for diabetic foot infections. Cochrane Database Syst Rev 2009;(3):CD006810.
38. Berlanga J, Fernandez JI, Lopez E, et al. Heberprot-P: a novel product for treating advanced diabetic foot ulcer. MEDICC Rev 2013;15(1):11–5.
39. Cohen IK, Crossland MC, Garrett A, et al. Topical application of epidermal growth factor onto partial-thickness wounds in human volunteers does not enhance reepithelialization. Plast Reconstr Surg 1995;96(2):251–4.
40. Hollier B, Harkin DG, Leavesley D, et al. Responses of keratinocytes to substrate-bound vitronectin: growth factor complexes. Exp Cell Res 2005;305(1):221–32.
41. Mishra S, Murphy LC, Nyomba BL, et al. Prohibitin: a potential target for new therapeutics. Trends Mol Med 2005;11(4):192–7.
42. Fernandez-Montequin JI, Valenzuela-Silva CM, Diaz OG, et al. Intra-lesional injections of recombinant human epidermal growth factor promote granulation and healing in advanced diabetic foot ulcers: multicenter, randomised, placebo-controlled, double-blind study. Int Wound J 2009;6(6):432–43.

43. Fernandez-Montequin JI, Betancourt BY, Leyva-Gonzalez G, et al. Intralesional administration of epidermal growth factor-based formulation (Heberprot-P) in chronic diabetic foot ulcer: treatment up to complete wound closure. Int Wound J 2009;6(1):67–72.

44. Alvarez Duarte H, Fors Lopez MM, Carretero JH, et al. Tolerability and safety of conventional therapy combination with DeMarco formula for infected ischemic diabetic foot. J Tissue Viability 2010;19(3):116–22.

45. Koenig W. Fibrin(ogen) in cardiovascular disease: an update. Thromb Haemost 2003;89(4):601–9.

46. Ehrly AM. Influence of urokinase on the flow properties of blood (Abstract). Clin Hemorheol 1985;5:728.

47. Weck M, Rietzsch H, Lawall H, et al. Intermittent intravenous urokinase for critical limb ischemia in diabetic foot ulceration. Thromb Haemost 2008;100(3): 475–82.

48. McGowan MP. Emerging low-density lipoprotein (LDL) therapies: management of severely elevated LDL cholesterol-The role of LDL-apheresis. J Clin Lipidol 2013;7(Suppl 3):S21–6.

49. Walzl M, Walzl B, Haas A. Heparin-induced extracorporeal fibrinogen/LDL precipitation (HELP): a promising regimen for the treatment of vascular diseases. Angiology 1997;48(12):1031–6.

50. Rietzsch H, Panzner I, Selisko T, et al. Heparin-induced Extracorporal LDL precipitation (H.E.L.P) in diabetic foot syndrome - preventive and regenerative potential? Horm Metab Res 2008;40(7):487–90.

51. Frykberg RG. Team approach toward lower extremity amputation prevention in diabetes. J Am Podiatr Med Assoc 1997;87(7):305–12.

52. Kawamura A, Horie T, Tsuda I, et al. Prevention of limb amputation in patients with limbs ulcers by autologous peripheral blood mononuclear cell implantation. Ther Apher Dial 2005;9(1):59–63.

53. Vojtassak J, Danisovic L, Kubes M, et al. Autologous biograft and mesenchymal stem cells in treatment of the diabetic foot. Neuro Endocrinol Lett 2006; 27(Suppl 2):134–7.

54. Gabr H, Hedayet A, Imam U, et al. Limb salvage using intramuscular injection of unfractionated autologous bone marrow mononuclear cells in critical limb ischemia: a prospective pilot clinical trial. Exp Clin Transplant 2011;9(3): 197–202.

Imaging of Diabetic Foot Infections

Robert Fridman, DPM[a],*, Tzvi Bar-David, DPM[a],
Stewart Kamen, DPM[a], Ronald B. Staron, MD[b],
David K. Leung, MD, PhD[b], Michael J. Rasiej, MD[b]

KEYWORDS

- Diabetic foot osteomyelitis • Diabetes • Infections • Imaging

KEY POINTS

- It is imperative that the clinician makes a quick and successful diagnosis of diabetic foot infection because a delay in treatment may lead to worsening outcomes.
- Imaging studies aid in the diagnosis of diabetic foot infections, particularly osteomyelitis.
- There are several mimickers of diabetic foot osteomyelitis, particularly neuroarthropathy, which may present difficulties in making a correct diagnosis.

INTRODUCTION

Complications from diabetic foot infections are a leading cause of nontraumatic lower-extremity amputations.[1] Nearly 85% of all of these amputations are a result of an infected foot ulcer.[2] Osteomyelitis (OM) is present in approximately 20% of diabetic foot infections.[3] Lavery and colleagues[4] reported a significant increase in the likelihood of lower-extremity amputation in patients with diabetic foot OM (DFO). Mutluoglu and colleagues[5] compared a group of patients with DFO versus soft tissue infection alone and concluded that the presence of OM negatively affects both the treatment and outcome of diabetic foot infections. It is, therefore, imperative that the clinician makes a quick and successful diagnosis of DFO because a delay in treatment may lead to worsening outcomes.[6] Imaging studies, such as plain films, bone scans, musculoskeletal ultrasound, computerized tomography (CT) scans, magnetic resonance imaging (MRI), and positron emission tomography scans, aid in the diagnosis. However, there are several mimickers of DFO, particularly neuroarthropathy, which present problems to making a correct diagnosis.[7,8]

[a] Division of Podiatric Surgery, Department of Orthopaedic Surgery, Columbia University Medical Center, New York, NY, USA; [b] Department of Radiology, Columbia University Medical Center, New York, NY, USA
* Corresponding author. 60 East 56th Street, New York, NY 10022.
E-mail address: RF2256@columbia.edu

Clin Podiatr Med Surg 31 (2014) 43–56
http://dx.doi.org/10.1016/j.cpm.2013.09.002
0891-8422/14/$ – see front matter © 2014 Elsevier Inc. All rights reserved.
podiatric.theclinics.com

PLAIN RADIOGRAPHS

A conventional radiograph is usually the first screening modality used for suspected diabetic foot infection. It is relatively inexpensive, noninvasive, and easily obtainable, often in the physician's own office. It provides an overview of the anatomy and may suggest the correct diagnosis, exclude other diagnostic possibilities, or provide clues for underlying pathologic conditions.[9] Cellulitis may be seen as nonspecific soft tissue thickness and opacity (**Fig. 1**).[10]

Life-threatening soft tissue infections, such as gas gangrene and necrotizing fasciitis, may present as radiolucent gas bubbles in the subcutaneous tissues on plain films, warranting immediate surgical intervention (**Fig. 2**).[11,12]

Acute OM is associated with inflammatory bone changes caused by pathogenic bacteria and is visible as demineralization, periosteal reaction, and osseous destruction (**Fig. 3**).[13] This process usually takes about 2 weeks to present after bone infection, when 30% to 50% of the bone mineral content has been lost,[9] which delays the diagnosis.

Additionally, plain films lack specificity for OM. False-positive diagnoses of OM may reflect neuroarthropathic changes in the absence of infection, yet may be interpreted as infectious processes, such as osteolysis or septic arthritis (**Fig. 4**).[14] Dinh[15] performed a meta-analysis on the diagnostic accuracy of plain films on DFO and found it to be of low to moderate accuracy. Newman and colleagues[3] reported on a series of 25 patients (41 diabetic foot ulcers) who had a 28% radiographic diagnosis of OM and bone biopsy and culture, which was 68% positive. An early report by Yuh[16] comparing plain films, bone scintigraphy, and MRI diagnoses with bone cultures had a 75% sensitivity and specificity for OM. Shults[17] reported a sensitivity of 52% sensitivity and 67% specificity for OM and recommended not using plain films as the sole diagnostic indicator for antibiotic or surgical intervention.

MUSCULOSKELETAL ULTRASOUND

Musculoskeletal ultrasound (MSK-US) is noninvasive and readily available but has limited uses when dealing with diabetic foot infections.[18] An abscess is visualized as fluid containing multiple internal echoes, which moves and swirls on compression, as compared with simple fluid, which appears hypoechoic or black with an absence of echoes.[10] MSK-US is helpful in the localization of foreign bodies and guidance for the needle aspiration of abscesses or collections.[19] If pathologic conditions of a tendon is suspected, real-time assessment of tendon integrity can be determined with active movement of the tendon. In cases of complete tendon rupture, the retracted tendon ends can be identified preoperatively.[18]

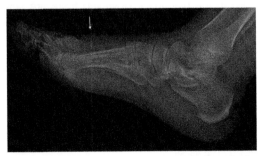

Fig. 1. The lateral radiograph of the foot shows non-specific soft tissue swelling (*arrow*) visible dorsally as thickening of the soft tissues.

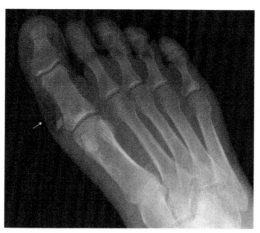

Fig. 2. Dorsoplantar radiographic view shows gas in the soft tissues, visible as small dark areas (*arrow*), around the radio-opaque foreign body that is visible as a sharply angulated density near the first metatarsal head.

RADIONUCLIDE BONE SCANS

Bone scans use labeled radiotracers to identify sites of active bone formation and are helpful in diagnosing OM. The most commonly used radiotracers are the technetium-99m labeled bisphosphonates, such as Tc-99m methylene diphosphonate (MDP) and Tc-99m hydroxy diphosphonate. Tracer uptake depends on blood flow and new regional osteoblastic activity.[20] For diagnosing OM, a 3-phase bone scan is typically performed. The initial angiogram or blood flow phase is acquired immediately after tracer bolus and consists of serial 1- to 5-second images of the area. The blood-pooling phase is performed 5 minutes after radiotracer injection. In areas of soft tissue inflammation, such as infection, capillaries will dilate, causing increased blood flow

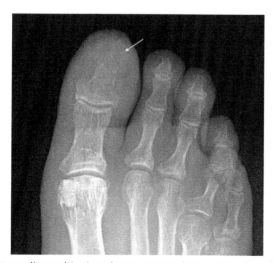

Fig. 3. Dorsoplantar radiographic view shows osseous destruction of the first distal phalanx (*arrow*), visible as deficiency of the bone of the distal tuft, indicating acute osteomyelitis.

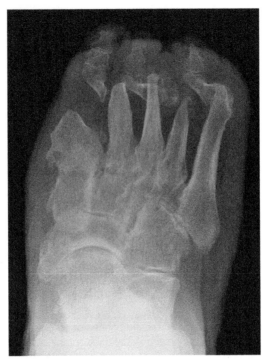

Fig. 4. Dorsoplantar radiographic view shows atrophic neuropathic changes with multiple areas of osseous deficiency in the forefoot.

and blood pooling. The third part, known as the delayed or bone phase, is performed 3 to 5 hours later. In cases of cellulitis, uptake occurs in the first 2 phases, but uptake is normal or diffusely increased in the third phase.[21]

The classic appearance of OM on 3-phase bone imaging is focal hyperperfusion in phase 1 indicating hyperemia, soft tissue inflammation in phase 2, and focal bone localization in phase 3 (**Fig. 5**). Bone scans are highly sensitive and can be positive as early as 2 days after the onset of symptoms.[22] However, because osteogenesis is a nonspecific response to stimuli, there are a host of reasons a bone scan may be positive, including physiologic growth, mechanical stress on bone, injury to bone, increased blood flow, tumors, and infection.[23] Bone scans are rarely false positive and, therefore, may be useful in determining if a foreign body penetrated bone because a negative result can be interpreted as no bone involvement.

Radionuclide techniques for imaging infection have vastly improved with the introduction of in vitro labeled leukocytes, such as indium-111 oxyquinoline and technetium-99m-hexamethylpropyleneamine oxime. An absolute white blood cell count of at least 2000/μL is needed to appropriately visualize any infection. A blood draw is performed, and the neutrophils are tagged with a radiotracer. Because most bacterial infections are mediated with a neutrophil inflammatory response, an increase in radiotracer signifies likely infection in the area. However, labeled leukocytes do accumulate naturally in the bone marrow of normal adults, which may confound results. Therefore, it is, at times, necessary to perform technetium-99m sulfur colloid marrow imaging in conjunction with labeled leukocyte imaging[24] but typically not essential in distal extremities. Both labeled leukocytes and sulfur colloid accumulate in the bone marrow, but sulfur colloid does not accumulate in areas of infection.

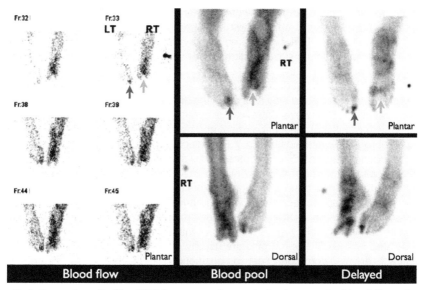

Fig. 5. A three phase Tc-99m DMP bone scan demonstrates hyperemia (blood flow phase) and soft tissue inflammation (blood pool phase) involving the right midfoot and left hallux (*arrows*). On the delayed images, radiotracer accumulates in the left hallux (*red arrow*), indicating osteomyelitis. However, the radiotracer uptake has resolved on the right (*green arrow*), indicating cellulitis without underlying osteomyelitis in the right midfoot.

The collective study is positive for infection when there is activity on the labeled leukocyte image and no activity on the sulfur colloid marrow image. Palestro and colleagues[25] reported that the overall accuracy of combined leukocyte-marrow imaging is approximately 90%.

MRI

MRI has been shown to be very sensitive in detecting cellulitis, soft tissue abscesses, and OM.[26] Croll and colleagues[27] evaluated the accuracy, sensitivity, and specificity of MRI, plain radiography, and nuclear scanning for diagnosing OM and concluded that MRI seemed to be the single best test for identifying bone infection. MRI uses the body's natural magnetic properties to help produce detailed anatomic images. The single-proton hydrogen nucleus is used for imaging purposes because it is found in large quantities in both fat and water in the body.[28] During an examination, an MRI magnet aligns the average magnetic moment of hydrogen protons in a given area along an axis and creates a magnetic vector. As a radiofrequency wave is added to the magnetic field, it deflects the magnetic vector. When the radiofrequency wave is turned off, the magnetic vector (measured as T1 relaxation) and axial spins of the hydrogen molecules (measured as T2 relaxation) return to their resting state, creating measurable signals that are translated into images.[28] Most pathologic conditions, including skin and bone infections, have a marked increase in water content; it is for this reason that MRI is very sensitive in disease detection.[27]

Standard variations in imaging parameters, such as echo time and repetition time, allow optimal visualization of relevant anatomy and aid in the recognition of pathologic conditions. In a T1-weighted image, fat appears brighter than water, and both normal and abnormal anatomy is well delineated. In T2-fat saturated sequences, water appears bright, and edema and inflammatory changes are optimally visualized.[29] In addition to T2-fat saturated sequences, short tau inversion recovery (STIR) images are also sensitive to slight changes in water content of bone marrow caused by OM.[10]

Infusion of intravenous gadolinium contrast may help demonstrate sinus tracts and abscesses more readily and may also aid in the differentiation of viable from nonviable bone or soft tissue.[30] However, intravenous contrast is contraindicated in patients with diabetes with significant renal impairment and must be weighed against the potential risk of nephrogenic systemic fibrosis.[10] In addition, ischemic tissue may show altered contrast uptake patterns,[30] with postsurgical changes and trauma causing false-positive results.[31,32] Therefore, gadolinium should be reserved for when there is suspected infection in or around a joint or possible abscess formation.[33]

Skin ulcerations appear as defects in the cutaneous line on MRI. Cellulitis and associated soft tissue edema is often seen in close proximity to an ulcer and manifests as a decrease of the normally high T1 signal intensity of fat and as a high signal on T2-weighted images.[34] The margins are usually poorly defined in cellulitis (**Fig. 6**).[29] Sinus tracts are also commonly seen in conjunction with ulcers and OM. Postcontrast fat-suppressed T1-weighted images are helpful to differentiate sinus tracts from adjacent soft tissue edema.[28] Abscess has been reported on MRI from 10% to 50% in patients with diabetic foot infections.[31,35] It is visualized as a fluidlike collection on T2 or STIR images, with a thick rim of enhancement postcontrast.[36]

Clinical suspicion for OM is increased when there is marrow edema in a bone within the vicinity of an ulceration.[37] Acute OM demonstrates confluent medullary hypointensity of the bone marrow on T1-weighted images and increased signal intensity on T2-weighted fat-suppressed images. Reactive marrow edema seen as a high T2-weighted fat-suppressed signal without corresponding confluent low T1 signal does not indicate OM (**Fig. 7**).[38] Periostitis is visible as a thin, linear pattern of edema with enhancement of the outer cortical bone (**Fig. 8**).[29] In acute OM, periostitis may be visible within the first few hours of infection on MRI, which is significantly quicker than changes seen on conventional radiographs, which may take up to 2 weeks to develop.[26]

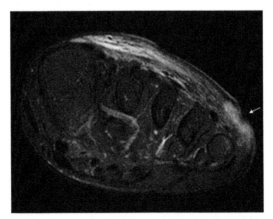

Fig. 6. An axial T2-weighted fat suppressed image of the forefoot shows an ulcer overlying the distal fifth metatarsal, visible as a superficial soft tissue indentation and discontinuity of the skin line (arrow), with an area of relatively bright signal underlying the ulcer indicating cellulitis. There is no osteomyelitis in the underlying bone.

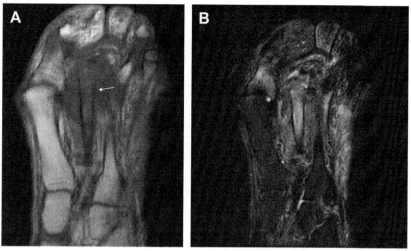

Fig. 7. Coronal T1-weighted (*A*) and Inversion Recovery (*B*) images of the forefoot show osteomyelitis of the second metatarsal visible as confluent low T1 bone marrow (*arrow*) and markedly higher signal than normal on the Inversion Recovery image (*arrow*).

One of the most useful applications of MRI is in the differentiation of infection from neuroarthropathy, which is commonly seen in patients with diabetes. Neuroarthropathy is the result of constant, repetitive trauma to joints in patients with peripheral neuropathy and peripheral vascular disease (PVD).[29] The neuropathy is responsible for

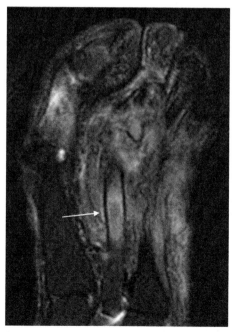

Fig. 8. A coronal Inversion Recovery image of the same forefoot as **Figure 7** shows a thin line of periostitis along the medial aspect of the second metatarsal diaphysis that is visible as a very thin line of high signal parallel to the dark line of the medial bone cortex (*arrow*).

Table 1
Stages on neuroarthropathy

Stage	Radiograph Features	MRI Features	Clinical Features
0: Incipient bone and joint damage	Widening of joint spaces, mild osteoarthrosis, or normal bone anatomy	Bone edema, bone bruise, stress fractures without cortical disruption, soft tissue edema, joint subluxation, cartilage damage, joint effusion	Swelling, erythema, warmth
I: Bone resorption	Widening of joint spaces, mild osteoarthrosis, or normal bone anatomy	Bone edema, bone bruise, fractures with cortical disruption, osteonecrosis, joint subluxation, soft tissue edema, joint effusion, foot deformity	More swelling, erythema, warmth, minor bone deformity, joint instability
II: Bone coalescence	Remineralization of regional bone, absorption of osseous debris, callous formation, adherence and coalescence of bone fragments, joint dislocations, foot deformity	Less bone edema, less bone bruise, less soft tissue edema, less joint effusion, joint subluxation, callus formation, foot deformity	Less swelling, less erythema, less warmth, major bone deformity, joint instability
III: Bone remodeling	Osteoarthrosis, joint space collapse, joint subluxation, subchondral erosions, sclerosis, fibrous ankylosis, rounding and smoothing of bone fragments, foot deformity	Osteoarthrosis, subchondral erosions, joint subluxation, narrowing of joint spaces, (residual bone edema, joint effusion), foot deformity	No swelling, no erythema, no warmth, fixed bone deformity, joint stiffness

From Chantelau E. Evaluation of the diabetic Charcot foot by MR imaging or plain radiography–an observational study. Exp Clin Endocrinol Diabetes 2006;114(8):428–31; with permission.

decreased sensitivity to trauma, and the ischemia from PVD results in poor bone healing, joint instability, deformity, and increased new bone formation.[29] This disease is usually seen in the midfoot and the tarsometatarsal joints. As the disease progresses, there is collapse of the arch, increased weight bearing on the cuboid, and a rocker-bottom appearance of the foot.[39] Neuroarthropathy is present in acute and chronic variations and may be staged as depicted in **Table 1**.[40] Stage 0 neuroarthropathy, as described by Yu and Hudson,[41] can only be appreciated with MRI because these initial changes are not visible on plain-film radiographs. Early neuroarthropathy may mimic OM because they both demonstrate high signal on T2 and STIR images and low T1 signal (**Fig. 9**). The clinical appearance of the foot must also be appreciated because OM is usually found in feet with open wounds, whereas neuroarthropathy has edematous, yet intact skin. MRI findings should always be coupled with clinical findings to achieve an accurate diagnosis. **Table 2** demonstrates some radiographic features of both OM and neuroarthropathy on MRI.[29]

CT

CT scans may be beneficial in identifying focal changes to infected bone, such as sequestra, cortical destruction, and periostitis.[42] However, CT scans cannot distinguish between purulence, granulation tissue, inflammation, and fibrosis.[42] It is, therefore, not a recommended solitary modality for imaging of diabetic foot infection if other

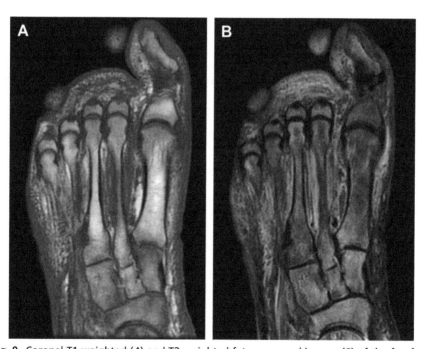

Fig. 9. Coronal T1-weighted (*A*) and T2-weighted fat suppressed images (*B*) of the forefoot show diffuse bone marrow edema, visible as slightly lower than normal signal within the marrow of the visualized bones on the T1-weighted image and brighter than normal signal on the T2-weighted image. There is also tissue edema as a result of neuroarthropathy that is visible on the T2-weighted image as streaky bright signal throughout the soft tissues and in the muscles between the bones.

Table 2
Differentiation of OM and neuroarthropathy on MRI

	OM	Neuroarthropathy
Bone marrow signal change	Low signal on T1 High signal on T2 and STIR	Acute: similar appearance to OM Chronic: normal or low T1 and T2
Bone marrow edema pattern	Involves solitary bone with diffuse bone marrow involvement	Periarticular and subchondral
Distribution	Focal	Multiple bones and joints
Location	Weight-bearing areas: toes, metatarsal head, protrusions, heel	Midfoot, tarsometatarsal joints
Deformity	Rare	Common
Soft tissue changes	Accompanies ulcer, sinus tract, or abscess	Intact but with edema

Adapted from Tan PL, The J. MRI of the diabetic foot: differentiation of infection from neuropathic change. Br J Radiol 2007;80:939–48.

modalities, such as MRI or scintigraphy, are available.[43,44] CT scan may be useful in detecting soft tissue gas, if present, in necrotizing fasciitis; however, imaging should not delay surgical management of this life-threatening infection.[45] Necrotizing fasciitis is seen on CT as fat stranding, along with fluid and gas collections that dissect along fascial planes.[46]

SINGLE-PHOTON EMISSION CT/CT

Scintigraphic studies are limited in exactly locating a focus of infection because of a lack of anatomic specificity and low resolution.[47] Combining scintigraphic images with an anatomic study at the same session using hybrid single-photon emission

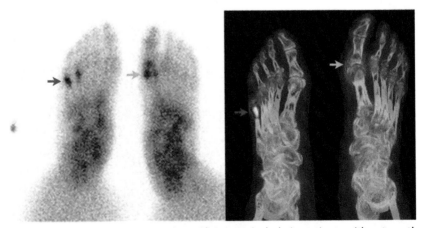

Fig. 10. MDP bone scans have limited specificity particularly in patients with osteoarthrosis and other conditions. On the planar image (*left*) both the right fifth and left first toes demonstrate focal accumulation of radiotracer (*arrows*) in the three-phase bone scan. Fusion SPECT-CT MIP image (*right*) increases the specificity, allowing clear-cut differentiation of osteomyelitis involving the distal diaphysis of the right fifth metatarsal (*red arrow*) from degenerative changes at the left first metatarsophalangeal joint (*green arrow*).

CT/CT (SPECT/CT) was introduced to overcome this challenge. This technique provides a fusion image with precise functional-anatomic correlation.[48] The current protocols call for either MDP injection (**Fig. 10**) or leukocyte labeling (**Fig. 11**) with subsequent planar scans (for leukocyte scans, at 30 minutes, 4 hours, and 24 hours after administration), with SPECT/CT image gathering at 4 to 6 hours.[48] In a study conducted by Filippi,[48] SPECT/CT changed the interpretation of 52% of images (10 of 19 suspected sites) when planar and SPECT images were performed alone. Horger and colleagues[49] showed that SPECT/CT enabled the distinction between soft tissue and bone infections in chronic OM better than SPECT alone, with specificity 89% on SPECT/CT versus 78% on SPECT. Sensitivity was identical for both SPECT and SPECT/CT at 100%. Heiba and colleagues[50] recommend the use of dual-isotope SPECT/CT imaging over single-isotope SPECT/CT alone because it considerably increased diagnostic accuracy.[50]

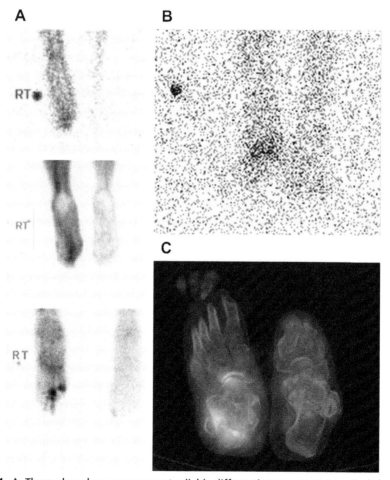

Fig. 11. A. Three phase bone scan cannot reliably differentiate recent postsurgical changes from osteomyelitis. B. In-111 labeling leukocyte differentiates right midfoot infection from postsurgical changes the right first and second toes, but with poor anatomical correlation. C. Fusion leukocyte SPECT/CT increases specificity as well as anatomical details.

REFERENCES

1. Boulton AJ, Vileikyte L, Ragnarson-Tennvall G, et al. The global burden of diabetic foot disease. Lancet 2005;366:1719–24.
2. Lipsky BA. Osteomyelitis of the foot in diabetic patients. Clin Infect Dis 1997;25: 1318–26.
3. Newman LG, Waller J, Palestro CJ, et al. Unsuspected osteomyelitis in diabetic foot ulcers. Diagnosis and monitoring by leukocyte scanning with indium in 111 oxyquinoline. JAMA 1991;266:1246–51.
4. Lavery LA, Armstrong DG, Wunderlich RP, et al. Risk factors for foot infections in individuals with diabetes. Diabetes Care 2006;29(6):1288–93.
5. Mutluoglu M, Sivrioglu AK, Eroglu M, et al. The implications of the presence of osteomyelitis on outcomes of infected diabetic foot wounds. Scand J Infect Dis 2013;45(7):497–503.
6. Sia I. Infection and musculoskeletal conditions: osteomyelitis. Best Pract Res Clin Rheumatol 2006;20:1065–81.
7. Berendt A. Diabetic foot osteomyelitis: a progress report on diagnosis and a systematic review of treatment. Diabetes Metab Res Rev 2008;24(Suppl 1): S145–61.
8. Baker J. Diabetic musculoskeletal complications and their imaging mimics. Radiographics 2012;32:1959–74.
9. Pineda C, Espinosa R, Pena A. Radiographic imaging in osteomyelitis: the role of plain radiography, computed tomography, ultrasonography, magnetic resonance imaging, and scintigraphy. Semin Plast Surg 2009;23(2):80–9.
10. Loredo RA, Rahal A, Garcia G, et al. Imaging of the diabetic foot diagnostic dilemmas. Foot Ankle Spec 2010;3:249–64.
11. Fisher JR, Conway MJ, Takeshita RT, et al. Necrotizing fasciitis. Importance of roentgenographic studies for soft-tissue gas. JAMA 1979;241:803–6.
12. Headley AJ. Necrotizing soft tissue infections: a primary care review. Am Fam Physician 2003;68:323–8.
13. Hatzenbuehler J, Pulling TJ. Diagnosis and management of osteomyelitis. Am Fam Physician 2011;84:1027–33.
14. Gold RH, Tong DJ, Crim JR, et al. Imaging the diabetic foot. Skeletal Radiol 1995;24(8):563–71.
15. Dinh M. Diagnostic accuracy of the physical examination and imaging tests for osteomyelitis underlying diabetic foot ulcers: meta-analysis. Clin Infect Dis 2008;47:519–27.
16. Yuh W. Osteomyelitis of the foot in diabetic patients: evaluation with plain film, 99mTc-MDP bone scintigraphy, and MR imaging. Am J Roentgenol 1989;152: 795–800.
17. Shults D. Value of radiographs and bone scans in determining the need for therapy in diabetic patients with foot ulcers. Am J Surg 1989;158:525–9 [discussion: 529–30].
18. Sanverdi S. Current challenges in imaging of the diabetic foot. Diabet Foot Ankle 2012;3:22.
19. Loredo RA, Garcia G, Chhaya S. Medical imaging of the diabetic foot. Clin Podiatr Med Surg 2007;24:397–424.
20. Love C. Radionuclide imaging of inflammation and infection in the acute care setting. Semin Nucl Med 2013;43:102–13.
21. Schauwecker DS. The scintigraphic diagnosis of osteomyelitis. AJR Am J Roentgenol 1992;158(1):9–18.

22. Handmaker H, Leonards R. The bone scan in inflammatory osseous disease. Semin Nucl Med 1976;6:95–105.
23. Mettler FA Jr, Guiberteau MJ. Essentials of nuclear medicine imaging. 6th edition. Philadelphia: Elsevier; 2012.
24. Palestro CJ, Love C, Miller TT. Infection and musculoskeletal conditions: imaging of musculoskeletal infections. Best Pract Res Clin Rheumatol 2006;20(6): 1197–218.
25. Palestro CJ, Love C, Tronco GG, et al. Combined labeled leukocyte and technetium-99m sulfur colloid marrow imaging for diagnosing musculoskeletal infection: principles, technique, interpretation, indications and limitations. Radiographics 2006;26:859–70.
26. Rosenberg ZS, Beltran J, Bencardino JT. MR imaging of the ankle and foot. Radiographics 2000;(20 Spec No):S153–79.
27. Croll SD, Nicholas GG, Osborne MA, et al. Role of magnetic resonance imaging in the diagnosis of osteomyelitis in diabetic foot infections. J Vasc Surg 1996;24: 266–70.
28. Berger A. Magnetic resonance imaging. BMJ 2002;324(7328):35.
29. Tan PL, The J. MRI of the diabetic foot: differentiation of infection from neuropathic change. Br J Radiol 2007;80:939–48.
30. Vartanians VM, Karchmer AW, Giurini JM, et al. Is there a role for imaging in the management of patients with diabetic foot? Skeletal Radiol 2009;38(7):633–6.
31. Unger E, Moldofsky P, Gatenby R, et al. Diagnosis of osteomyelitis by MR imaging. AJR Am J Roentgenol 1988;150(3):605–10.
32. Erdman WA, Tamburro F, Jayson HT, et al. Osteomyelitis: characteristics and pitfalls of diagnosis with MR imaging. Radiology 1991;180(8):533–9.
33. Miller TT, Randolph DA Jr, Staron RB, et al. Fat-suppressed MRI of musculoskeletal infection: fast T2-weighted techniques versus gadolinium-enhanced T1-weighted images. Skeletal Radiol 1997;26(11):654–8.
34. Marcus CD, Ladam-Marcus VJ, Leone J, et al. MR imaging of osteomyelitis and neuropathic osteoarthropathy in the feet of diabetics. Radiographics 1996; 16(6):1337–48.
35. Beltran J, Campanini DS, Knight C, et al. The diabetic foot: magnetic resonance imaging evaluation. Skeletal Radiol 1990;19:37–41.
36. Ledermann HP, Morrison WB, Schweitzer ME, et al. Tendon involvement in pedal infection: MR analysis of frequency, distribution, and spread of infection. AJR Am J Roentgenol 2002;179:939–47.
37. Tang JS, Gold RH, Bassett LW, et al. Musculoskeletal infection of the extremities: evaluation with MR imaging. Radiology 1988;166:205–9.
38. Collins MS, Schaar MM, Wenger DE, et al. T1-weighted MRI characteristics of pedal osteomyelitis. Am J Roentgenol 2005;185:386–93.
39. Armstrong DG, Lavery LA. Elevated peak plantar pressures in patients who have Charcot arthropathy. J Bone Joint Surg Am 1998;80(3):365–9.
40. Chantelau E. Evaluation of the diabetic Charcot foot by MR imaging or plain radiography–an observational study. Exp Clin Endocrinol Diabetes 2006; 114(8):428–31.
41. Yu GV, Hudson JR. Evaluation and treatment of stage 0 Charcot's neuroarthropathy of the foot and ankle. J Am Podiatr Med Assoc 2002;92:210–20.
42. Boutin RD, Brossman J, Sartoris DJ, et al. Update on imaging of orthopedic infections. Orthop Clin North Am 1998;29(1):41–66.
43. Sella E. Current concepts review: diagnostic imaging of the diabetic foot. Foot Ankle Int 2009;30:568–76.

44. Berquist TH, Brown ML, Fitzgerald R, et al. Magnetic resonance imaging: application in musculoskeletal infection. Magn Reson Imaging 1985;3:219–30.
45. Stoneback JW, Hak DJ. Diagnosis and management of necrotizing fasciitis. Orthopedics 2011;34(3):196.
46. Fayad LM, Carrino JA, Fishman EK. Musculoskeletal infection: role of CT in the emergency department. Radiographics 2007;27(6):1723–36.
47. Filippi L. Usefulness of hybrid SPECT/CT in 99mTc-HMPAO–Labeled leukocyte scintigraphy or bone and joint infections. J Nucl Med 2006;47:1908–13.
48. Filippi L. Diabetic foot infection: usefulness of SPECT/CT for 99mTc-HMPAO-labeled leukocyte imaging. J Nucl Med 2009;50:1042–6.
49. Horger M, Eschmann SM, Pfannenberg C, et al. The value of SPECT/CT in chronic osteomyelitis. Eur J Nucl Med Mol Imaging 2003;30:1665–73.
50. Heiba S, Kolker D, Mocherla B, et al. The optimized evaluation of diabetic foot infection by dual isotope SPECT/CT imaging protocol. J Foot Ankle Surg 2010; 49:529–36.

Current Therapies for Diabetic Foot Infections and Osteomyelitis

Bryan A. Sagray, DPM[a], Sabina Malhotra, DPM[b],
John S. Steinberg, DPM, FACFAS[c,d,*]

KEYWORDS

- Osteomyelitis • Diabetic foot • Infection • Abscess • Ischemia

KEY POINTS

- Diabetic Foot infections require rapid multidisciplinary team assessment.
- Use of bone culture, histology, and MRI is recommended, but osteomyelitis can be difficult to objectively diagnose.
- Spreading or deep diabetic foot infections likely require surgical inpatient management.
- The goal of therapy is to prevent amputation and to preserve as much of the weigh bearing surface as possible.
- Thorough vascular assessment and liberal revascularization are imperative to a successful outcome in treating a diabetic foot infection.

INTRODUCTION

The prevalence of diabetes continues to be a growing problem throughout the developed world and contributes significantly to the health care burden. Infections in the diabetic foot are often complicated by numerous other medical comorbidities, which can rapidly progress to major limb loss. Diabetic neuropathy, peripheral vascular disease, coronary artery disease, and end-stage renal disease on hemodialysis routinely accompany the patient with diabetes with lower extremity infection. Therefore, the recognition of non–limb-threatening versus limb-threatening infections is paramount in the patient with diabetes, facilitating a prompt treatment protocol.

Expert opinion and anecdotal evidence often determine how patients are treated, misleading the medical community and not allowing for a consensus on therapy. This may explain why numerous societies and organizations have been specifically established to address this concern and are continuing to update their recommendations regarding diabetic foot infections (DFIs). Prime examples include the Infectious

[a] The Permanente Medical Group, Department of Orthopaedics, Modesto/Stockton, California, USA; [b] San Diego, California; [c] Georgetown University School of Medicine, 3800 Reservoir Road, Northwest, Washington, DC 20007, USA; [d] Department of Plastic Surgery, Center for Wound Healing, MedStar Georgetown University Hospital, 3800 Reservoir Road, Northwest, Washington DC 20007, USA
* Corresponding author.
E-mail address: jss5@gunet.georgetown.edu

Clin Podiatr Med Surg 31 (2014) 57–70
http://dx.doi.org/10.1016/j.cpm.2013.09.003
0891-8422/14/$ – see front matter © 2014 Elsevier Inc. All rights reserved.

Diseases Society of America (IDSA) and the International Working Group on the Diabetic Foot (IWGDF). These two organizations strive to provide treatment protocols and guidelines specific to the DFI, stemming from evidence-based medicine.

STATISTICS AND RECENT DEVELOPMENTS

Recent literature has shed light on the complex pathology of DFIs. Subsequently, health care providers now have a better understanding as to why these infections are so prevalent, severe, and often difficult to treat. To a varying extent, the pathology of DFI involves the host and the bacteria. Host-related disturbances include immunopathy, neuropathy, and angiopathy. Several innate immunologic defects have been reported in patients with diabetes, such as impaired phagocytosis and bactericidal activity.[1] Pathogen density and virulence also play a role accounting for the severity of DFI. Recognizing these intricacies is imperative to the accurate diagnosis and treatment of DFIs and osteomyelitis.

DIAGNOSIS, IMAGING MODALITIES, AND RELATED CONTROVERSIES

DFIs are estimated to be the most common cause of diabetes-related hospital admissions and remain one of the major pathways to lower-limb amputation. In 2012, the IWGDF reported that every year, more than 1 million people with diabetes lose a leg as a consequence of this disease.[2] A foot ulcer precedes most of these amputations; once an ulcer has developed, infection and peripheral arterial disease are the major causes for amputation. Thus, the first step of diagnosis is crucial to ensuring swift recognition and management of an infection.

Infection is best defined as invasion and multiplication of microorganisms in host tissues that induces an inflammatory response in said host. This is usually followed by tissue destruction. DFIs are clinically defined as soft tissue or bone infections anywhere below the level of malleoli.[3,4]

Because all skin wounds harbor superficial microorganisms, their mere presence cannot provide evidence of infection. Recent reports suggest that greater than or equal to 10^5 colony-forming units of bacteria per gram of tissue can be used to quantify the presence of soft tissue infection.[5] However, it is nearly impossible to confirm such numbers in a diabetic foot ulcer outside of a research laboratory. Imaging techniques, such as plain film radiographs, ultrasound, and magnetic resonance imaging, are also limited and nonspecific for soft tissue infections. As such, the IDSA and IWGDF have jointly developed a clinical classification system for defining the presence and severity of a DFI.[3,4] According to these guidelines, clinical diagnosis is vested in the presence of at least two local findings of inflammation: redness, warmth, pain and tenderness, induration, and purulent secretions. Secondary features of suggested soft tissue infection include necrosis, friable granulation tissue, foul odor, or chronicity of wound and failure to heal within an expected timeline. As always, diabetic foot ulcers should be carefully and consistently inspected, palpated, and probed to assess for infection.

A bone infection should be suspected in two main situations: when an ulcer, usually overlying a bony prominence, fails to heal despite adequate treatment methods; and when a digit is uncharacteristically swollen, erythematous, and/or indurated (commonly referred to as a "sausage toe"). The clinical presentation of a bone infection in the diabetic foot can vary depending on the site involved, extent of infected bone, associated soft tissue involvement, causative organism, and adequacy of limb perfusion.[6]

Definitively diagnosing osteomyelitis in the clinical setting has recently become a topic of controversy. In 1995, Grayson and colleagues[7] introduced the "probe-to-bone test" (PTB) as a novel method for diagnosing diabetic foot osteomyelitis. Striking bone with a blunt sterile metal probe that is gently inserted through an ulcer indicates a positive test and an increased likelihood of osteomyelitis. Although this simple, quick, and inexpensive method has since gained wide acceptance, several investigators have recently questioned its validity and accuracy. A mainstay criticism of the original study is that Grayson and colleagues based their results on a hospitalized patient population with an already high prevalence of osteomyelitis (66%). Shone and colleagues[8] and Lavery and colleagues[9] undertook the same study on unselected outpatient populations with 23.5% and 12% of osteomyelitis prevalence, respectively. These authors found very low positive predictive values for the PTB test originally outlined by Grayson and colleagues. In contrast, they did find high negative predictive values, suggesting a negative PTB test in a patient at low risk for osteomyelitis essentially rules out infection.[3,4]

Most recently, Mutluoglu and colleagues[10] conducted a PTB study including outpatients and inpatients to specifically evaluate the diagnostic predictivity of the PTB test in a selected subgroup of patients clinically suspected of having diabetic foot osteomyelitis. In this study, PTB test results were positive in 46.1% of patients. The positive predictive value for the PTB test was 87% and the negative predictive value was 62%. Because the correlation of positive PTB test is not strong, these authors suggest using additional diagnostic modalities.

When ordering blood tests on a patient, an elevated erythrocyte sedimentation rate and C-reactive protein can indicate acute osteomyelitis. Erythrocyte sedimentation rate and C-reactive protein are acute-phase proteins, which reflect a measure of the acute-phase response. The term "acute phase" refers to local and systemic events that accompany inflammation. An elevated white blood cell count may also indicate infection of either soft tissue or bone.

Obtaining wound cultures has also been a recent topic of controversy. For infected ulcers, current IDSA guidelines recommend that clinicians send appropriately obtained specimens for culture before starting empiric antibiotic therapy. Swab specimens are now preferably avoided altogether, especially of inadequately debrided ulcers, because they provide less accurate results and are often full of surface contaminants. IDSA guidelines recommend sending a specimen for culture and histopathology that is from deep tissue, obtained by biopsy or curettage after the wound has been cleansed and debrided. Specimens should be sent to the laboratory promptly in suitable sterile transport containers.

A plethora of imaging modalities exists to aid in the diagnosis of DFI. The initial imaging study obtained is plain film radiographs, preferably as soon as possible and of bilateral feet for comparison. However, a common problem in diagnosing osteomyelitis is the delay in detecting bony changes in early infection on plain radiographs. It is also often difficult to distinguish bony changes caused by infection from those related to, for example, Charcot neuro-osteoarthropathy. Magnetic resonance imaging has been found to be the most sensitive and specific means of diagnosing diabetic foot osteomyelitis.[11] Nuclear medicine techniques including bone scans (^{99m}Tc-methylene diphosphate) and radiolabelled white blood cell scans (^{99m}Technetium or ^{111}Indium) may also have high positive predictive values for osteomyelitis. A recent review concluded that among radionuclide procedures, radiolabelled white blood cell imaging is the best choice for evaluating diabetic foot osteomyelitis, with a sensitivity of 72% to 100% and specificity of 67% to 98%.[12] When other studies are unavailable or contraindicated in a patient, a recent prospective study has recommended a combination of computed tomography with positron emission tomography as highly sensitive for osteomyelitis.[13]

Although the toolbox of today's diagnostician seemingly overflows with laboratory markers and imaging studies, a bone biopsy is still the gold standard for confirming osteomyelitis in the diabetic foot. IWGDF guidelines state that current evidence supports evaluating a bone specimen as the best available diagnostic technique for diagnosing bone infection and providing reliable data on the responsible organisms and their antibiotic susceptibility profile.[3,4] However, recent investigators have called into question the objectivity and reliability of bone biopsy with respect to the diagnosis of diabetic foot osteomyelitis. In a 2011 study by Meyr and colleagues[14], four pathologists were asked to retrospectively review 39 consecutive tissue specimens and were informed only that these were "a specimen of bone taken from a diabetic foot to evaluate for osteomyelitis." The pathologists were kept unaware of the previous pathology reports and specific patient clinical characteristics. All four pathologists completely agreed on a primary diagnosis of osteomyelitis in 13 (33.33%) of the 39 specimens. A situation of clinically significant disagreement, or in which at least one pathologist diagnosed "no evidence of OM," but at least one other pathologist diagnosed "findings consistent with OM," occurred in 16 (41.03%) of the specimens. The authors state these results emphasize the need for a more comprehensive diagnostic protocol for diabetic foot osteomyelitis. That being said, current IDSA guidelines suggest that the most definitive way to diagnose osteomyelitis in the diabetic foot is by the combined findings on bone culture and histology.

DECISION FOR NONOPERATIVE VERSUS OPERATIVE MANAGEMENT

Most DFIs require some degree of surgical intervention. These can range from minor (superficial debridement, incision and drainage, or excision of infected and necrotic tissues) to major (resections, reconstruction of soft tissue or bony defects, revascularization of the lower extremity, and lower limb amputations). In an early and evolving DFI, primary treatment modalities may entail localized superficial debridement, special dressing techniques, offloading, antibiotic therapy, and regimented follow-up on an outpatient basis. Conservative therapy may actually be preferred in this case as to avoid unnecessary surgical complications. An open dialogue should be maintained with the patient so that he or she is aware of the entire situation. An educated and motivated patient in combination with a supportive home environment can often spell the difference between successful outpatient therapy and the need for emergent hospitalization.

If a patient is unresponsive to conservative measures, or if the infection progresses, hospitalization is likely required for close monitoring and daily wound care. Extensive soft tissue cellulitis also warrants hospitalization for intravenous antibiotic therapy. According to current IDSA guidelines, urgent surgical intervention is required for most foot infections accompanied by gas in the deeper tissues, an abscess, or necrotizing fasciitis. Less urgent surgery is recommended for wounds with substantial nonviable tissue or extensive bone or joint involvement.[3,4] In the case of gas gangrene with pending sepsis, a decompression irrigation and drainage may be performed under local anesthesia until a more extensive surgical debridement can be performed. Any clinically suspected limb- or life-threatening infection should warrant urgent surgical consultation.

When addressing a patient's infection, the surgical approach used should optimize the likelihood for healing while attempting to preserve the integrity of the walking surface of the foot. The vascularity of the affected limb should also be evaluated, with referral to a vascular surgeon obtained as needed. Regardless of nonoperative versus operative management, appropriate wound care, antibiotic therapy, and regular outpatient follow-up are essential for successful cure of infection and subsequent healing of the wound.

SURGICAL APPROACH

After a decision is made for operative debridement of the DFI with concomitant osteomyelitis, many factors must be taken into consideration. Bone infection tends to accompany 50% to 60% of severe DFIs and 10% to 20% of the less severe.[15] Often these patients are medically unstable and present with complicating comorbidities. The presence of soft tissue gas/emphysema or necrotizing infection warrants urgent surgical intervention to prevent limb loss, potentially superseding medical optimization or revascularization. Examination of these particular patients requires an emphasis on the macrovascular arterial system, presence of palpable or dopplerable pulses, location of necrotic or devitalized tissue, and consideration for noninvasive arterial studies. However, moderate to severe infection presenting in the ischemic limb requires early discussion with vascular surgery or interventional radiology. Although the limb may not require urgent endovascular or traditional open bypass, consultation facilitates the well-recognized team approach to the diabetic foot.[16,17] After the spread of infection has been mitigated and the patient stabilized, the surgeon's ultimate goal should be preservation of foot function and stability, while preventing further tissue loss and subsequent breakdown.

The anatomy of the foot is complex and unique primarily because of its division into separate compartments.[18] These restrictive anatomic compartments can promote the spread of infection in one direction, while containing it into another. For example, deep infections within the plantar aspect of the foot can spread by way of the long flexors tendons to the deep posterior compartment of the lower leg.[18-21] On the contrary, containment of infection within a dorsal foot fascial compartment can increase local pressure and lead to tissue necrosis.[18-21] Ultimately, infection in the diabetic foot travels based on anatomic location, tendons within that compartment, point of entry, and type of organisms present.[22] Therefore, the treating surgeon should have an in-depth working knowledge of the foot and ankle and be closely involved throughout the treatment process. This enables initial incision placement for adequate control of infection, while not compromising definitive closure and reconstructive options available.

The adequacy of blood flow and distal tissue perfusion is paramount to delivery of intravenous antibiotics and surgical wound healing. This is further appreciated by the concept of an angiosome, defined by Taylor and later popularized by Attinger, which delineates the anatomic block of tissue supplied by a source artery.[23-25] Their research and principles allow the skilled surgeon to place incisions in a manner not to further compromise already ischemic tissue. Ideally, surgical incisions should be placed along the border of two angiosomes or at glabrous skin junctions, allowing maximal blood flow from either side of the wound. The diabetic patient often suffers from multilevel infrapopliteal atherosclerosis, often resulting in occlusion of a main source artery.[26] These findings further complicate surgical planning when an occlusion is evident and advocate incision placement within the territory of the diseased vessel to minimize damage to the patent source artery or communicating choke vessels.[25]

After the patient's blood flow status has been adequately evaluated and a decision for incisional approach made, the operating surgeon must also determine when the ideal time is to culture the wound. There is clear evidence that superficial wound swabs yield little useful information, especially when there are no clinical signs of infection.[27] Numerous sources recommend that specimens for culture be obtained from deep tissue, using biopsy or curettage.[27,28] However, controversy exists regarding when to perform wound culture, with relation to predebridement or postdebridement in the operating room. The 2012 report from the IDSA clinical practice guidelines emphasizes cleansing and debridement of the wound before obtaining tissue for culture.[28] Furthermore, a recent meta-analysis demonstrates that superficial swab culture compared with deep tissue culture in lower extremity wounds found 49% sensitivity and 62% specificity identification of correct infectious organism.[29] When bone or bone fragments are palpable or visible within the wound, high consideration should also be given to concomitant osteomyelitis. Bone specimens should be sent for culture and histopathology, with care taken in proper handling and processing.

This combination of soft tissue and concomitant bone infection in the patient with diabetes significantly dictates surgical approach. The presence of osteomyelitis increases the chance for operative debridement, amputation, and possibility of prolonged antibiotic therapy.[30] Occurrence can range from 20% in mild to moderately infected wounds and upward of 50% to 60% in severely infected wounds.[31] The surgical plan should include soft tissue debridement and adequate resection of infected or necrotic bone to minimize repeat operative and anesthetic risks. Persistence of sepsis, contraindications to prolonged antibiotic therapy, progressive bony deterioration, and an ability to achieve a primarily closeable wound should promote osseous resection.[28–30] However, care must be taken to preserve a stable and functional foot without increasing the risk of transfer lesions. When soft tissue infection has been eradicated and infected or necrotic bone resected, the surgeon must determine the appropriate time and manner for definitive wound closure.

Numerous articles and textbooks have been written detailing reconstructive techniques for wound closure. A generalized overview with minimal detail is provided here. Often referred to as the plastic reconstructive ladder or elevator or more recently a pyramid, these surgical protocols dictate simple to complex options.[31–34] Certain factors must be taken into consideration when selecting the appropriate technique, from wound characteristics, vascular status, presence of underlying deformity, residual infection, to patient medical comorbidities.[35] Entire articles have been dedicated to complicating medical comorbidities, including controlled or uncontrolled diabetes mellitus, renal insufficiency with or without hemodialysis, malnutrition, tobacco usage, ability to off-load, obesity, and compliance issues.[35] Each of the previously mentioned conditions tends to negatively impact wound healing and must be thoroughly explored by the treating surgeon; however, their details are beyond the scope of this article. After the patient and wound defect have been optimized, attempt at closure should proceed from simple and straightforward to complex.[36,37]

Allowing a wound to epithelize by secondary intention can be a viable option when large granular defects are present or the patient is unsuited for further surgical or anesthetic associated risks. If the wound is amendable to primary closure and can be done so without undue tension, then low-reactive nonabsorbable sutures or staples should be considered, avoiding placement of deep highly reactive braided suture material. Another option for closure is split-thickness skin grafting (STSG) versus full-thickness skin grafting. Focus is placed on the STSG rather than the full-thickness skin grafting because they tend to have more application and reliability in reconstruction in the patient with diabetes. These particular grafts have wide versatility and can be applied over large granular wounds, dermal tissue, fascia, exposed muscle, or periosteum.[38,39] However, special care should be taken when considering application over large areas of exposed bone without intact periosteum or in plantar weight-bearing surfaces.[38,39] STSG should ideally be placed over wounds with granulation tissue, which tends to signify adequate perfusion and absence of bacterial contamination. Techniques for STSG fixation include absorbable or nonabsorbable suture, surgical staples, and platelet-rich plasma, with traditional tie-over bolster and recently negative pressure wound therapy for graft immobilization.[40,41] Local flaps are slightly more complex than skin grafting, but provide numerous advantages. Providing more bulk, local flaps are able to cover plantar weight-bearing surfaces, their dissection provides access to underlying structures preventing further incisions, and their native tissue vascularity is maintained. The vascular supply is either a cutaneous, musculocutaneous, or septocutaneous artery, making full-thickness dissection of the flap paramount. Tissue retraction and exposure should be gentle with sharp skin hooks; usage of loupe magnification is beneficial, as is intraoperative hand-held Doppler for perforator location. Because of the consistent vascular supply of the plantar foot, extensive undermining should be avoided when performing local random flap closure. The previously discussed principle of angiosomes and concept of choke vessels are required knowledge for the surgeon performing all reconstructive closure techniques, but are most crucial when using local flaps and the following more complex procedures. Postoperative flap monitoring becomes necessary with local flaps, with importance increasing with muscle, pedicle, or free tissue transfer closure. Muscle flaps are increasingly complex and provide yet another option for closure. Intrinsic muscles of the foot allow for plantar, medial, and lateral defects to be approached. Their use is especially beneficial when reconstructing large osseous defects after bone infection debridement, to provide increased vascularity and delivery of antibiotics, and for coverage of exposed surgical hardware.[42,43] Dissection and handling techniques of muscle flaps follows that of local random flaps, but with even more emphasis placed on intraoperative use of loupe magnification and hand-held Doppler for identification of the dominant arterial pedicle. Extensive vascular anatomy is warranted to allow for appropriate selection of a potential alternate or nondominant arterial pedicle, which may allow for less kinking during rotation of the muscle about its axis. Muscle flaps require tension-free in-setting and minimal suturing to the surrounding dermis or skin.[35] If the surgeon suspects tenuous perfusion, grafting over the muscle may be delayed until further success can be determined with postoperative monitoring. Finally, pedicle-style flaps are discussed as an option for complex closure. Pedicle flaps require dissection and identification of the neurovascular bundle that provides perfusion and nourishment to the tissue in question. The need for isolation of source or perforator vessels requires detailed anatomic knowledge and surgical experience; ligation of nondominant vessels is also sometimes necessary. Pedicle flaps can be planned with antegrade/anatomic or retrograde/reverse flow, depending on location of the recipient site or defect characteristics.[35] Harvest can include the overlying skin or be raised as an island to allow for coverage of defects distant from the donor site. The more complex the procedure chosen, the more likely it is that complications will arise. Venous congestion and partial-thickness necrosis are common, often requiring revisional procedures. Patient selection and appropriate preoperative optimization is key, with the surgeon benefiting from knowledge of techniques to deal with said complications. Certain precautions have been identified in numerous publications as reliable additions when performing pedicle-style flaps, including delayed in-setting of the flap, inclusion of at least two accompanying veins, use of intraoperative hand-held Doppler and loupe magnification, external fixation for off-loading or immobilization, avoiding closure over the neurovascular pedicle, close postoperative observation, and availability of medicinal leeches.[35,44–46] Free tissue transfer or microvascular anastomosis is not discussed because of the complexity and detail required for explanation. Additional, novel techniques for eradication of soft tissue and bone infection with management of dead space are discussed next.

NOVEL SURGICAL TECHNIQUES USING ANTIBIOTIC DELIVERY SYSTEMS

The treatment approach for severe soft tissue and bone infection in the diabetic foot continues to evolve, but the addition of absorbable or nonabsorbable antibiotic delivery systems tends to be underused at this time. The reason for this is likely attributed to surgeon experience or training and a lack of conclusive peer-reviewed evidence-based literature. However, the concept of antibiotic-impregnated systems has been around since the early 1970s, when Buchholz and Engelbrecht began using the cement to salvage infected total hip arthroplasties.[47,48] Several years later Klemm[49] applied the concept to the dead space after resection of osteomyelitic bone. Less than 25 years after their introduction in the literature, a US hospital survey of 336 institutions demonstrated 27% of them were using antibiotic-impregnated beads or polymethylmethacrylate (PMMA) cement.[50]

The primary benefit of implanted antibiotic devices is high levels of localized active antibiotic, while still minimizing toxic systemic side effects. The exact mechanism of release is poorly understood, but is likely a combination of diffusion and elution within the surrounding tissues. Routine laboratory antibiotic sensitivity testing to determine bacterial resistance uses minimum inhibitory concentrations greater than 4 μg/mL.[51] Several studies testing local wound concentrations of PMMA-impregnated cement have demonstrated levels of 20 to 200 mg/mL, substantially above the routine testing levels.[52] The specific types of antibiotics available are numerous and must meet specific criteria with relation to solubility, heat tolerance, and overall chemical properties. Bacterial resistance and sensitivity and potential patient allergies also come into play. There are also commercially prefabricated systems and numerous techniques for surgeon-created bead or spacer systems. The details of each type of antibiotic and its delivery system characteristics are beyond the scope of this article.

Besides their ability to provide bacteriostatic and bacteriocidal killing properties, implanted antibiotics also facilitate the process of soft tissue and osseous reconstruction. The insertion of the device maintains length and structural rigidity, allowing aggressive debridement of infected soft tissue and bone, while promoting a soft tissue sheath to allow for delayed bone grafting.[53,54] Another advantage of PMMA antibiotic-impregnated cement is the ability to provide high local levels of antibiosis independent of vascular supply, a factor that routinely limits intravenous usage in patients with severe peripheral vascular disease, atherosclerosis, or diabetes. Schade and Roukis[55] also mention the unique avascular osseous nature of the foot, with a large ratio of cortical to cancellous bone present, further reducing likelihood of appropriate circulating systemic antibiotic levels. In another study of 36 patients with severely ischemic foot infections, PMMA antibiotic beads were essential in reducing the presence of bacterial burden of polymicrobial origin despite compromised vascularity.[56]

The use of antibiotic-loaded cement implants shows improved eradication of osseous infection over surgical debridement and parenteral antibiotics alone. However, their use primarily for severe diabetic soft tissue infections or after transmetatarsal amputations remains controversial. Many authors have discouraged against their usage in soft tissue infection alone because they require subsequential removal. This additional operative procedure possesses its own anesthetic risk factors and further incision or dissection through a previously potential tenuous vascular region. Also, the implant itself could become a nidus for infection after it has released its antibacterial contents, albeit unlikely.[57] These theoretical risk factors can be mitigated by impregnating the antibiotic in an absorbable vehicle or scaffold, instead of the traditional PMMA cement. These devices have unique properties, but are typically made of absorbable calcium sulfate or phosphate powder or bioabsorbable sponges made of gelatin or collagen. Further benefits to these newer absorbable vehicles include wider range of acceptable antibiotics for impregnation, potentially less interference on fluoroscopy or radiography detail, possibility of fewer operative procedures thereby reducing hospital length of stay and overall cost, and ability to use directly for allograft bone augmentation. Despite the clear advantage of implanted antibiotic delivery systems, inpatient multidisciplinary medical management combined with culture-driven parenteral antibiotics is paramount.[55] The treating surgeon should have a clear understanding of the indications, fabrication, and application of impregnated implantable antibiotic delivery systems because they have clear advantages in the severely infected or ischemic diabetic foot.

OUTCOMES

There are obvious factors that affect the success rate of treatment in the diabetic foot. Often the true rates of success or failure are difficult to ascertain because studies have extremely variable patient populations and severity of infections. One particular meta-analysis quoted failure at 22.7% after reviewing 18 separate studies.[58] The presence of methicillin-resistant *Staphylococcus aureus*, fever on initial presentation, increased serum creatinine, prior hospitalizations for DFI, and gangrenous changes were all related to treatment failure.[59] Another study further delineated the outcomes when osteomyelitis accompanied soft tissue infection, resulting in more surgical procedures, longer antibiotic duration, increased time to wound healing, and prolonged hospital length of stay.[60] The exact measurement of treatment success is also difficult because the literature often considers limb salvage the ultimate goal. However, often these patients may have ischemic and a nonhealing diabetic foot ulcer, not a true soft tissue or bone infection. Extrapolating and interrupting the data then becomes confusing. Theoretically, for a patient to be categorized as limb salvage success, eradication of infection and wound healing has taken placed. A recent study looking at limb salvage and 5-year survival rate found a success of 84.9% and 86.8%, respectively.[61] Aggressive surgical debridement and partial foot amputations have also shown long-term limb salvage rates and reduction in number of repeat operative procedures. For example, although partial first ray resections can progress to transmetatarsal amputations, they are a good initial procedure in maintaining bipedal ambulation, lowering morbidity and mortality related to major transtibial amputation.[62]

Even a brief review of the extensive literature published on DFI and limb salvage reveals a pervasive emphasis on revascularization. The theme of appropriate vascular supply to the diabetic extremity is paramount; whether it is addressed before surgical debridement or after initial drainage of infection remains controversial. However, all agree that success rates are drastically improved when vascular surgeons or interventional radiologist are involved in the process. Once again multidisciplinary approaches to DFI and limb salvage reveal beneficial outcomes, thereby this should become the norm. In 2010 alone, almost 2 million Americans were newly diagnosed with diabetes mellitus, a number that will surely continue to increase and plague the health care system.[63] Developing an integrated, multispecialty protocol for the diabetic foot should be at the forefront of health care research and must be based on sound evidence-based medicine.

RECURRENCE OF INFECTION OR OSTEOMYELITIS

The most important reason behind an aggressive medical and surgical approach to DFI is to prevent recurrence or progression, leading to major limb loss. The ability to define recurrence of infection or osteomyelitis after completion of therapy is difficult because often there is no scientific way to determine if the new infection is related to residual bacterial presence or new organisms. For example, several articles attempt to discuss the progression of further operative procedures after partial first ray resection for diabetic foot, but whether this is truly a biomechanical issue or presence of residual infection is difficult to determine.[64] Bacteria can remain dormant and patients without signs of inflammation, even after what seems to be clinical resolution of infection.

Approximately 15% of patients with diabetes develop a foot ulceration that requires treatment; however, 84% of the time amputation is the final result of a nonhealed ulceration.[65] An obvious risk for recurrence of bone infection is development of a new wound following treatment, allowing direct extension of offending organisms to the underlying deep structures. A large study with 330 patients with diabetes with osteomyelitis and 1808 without osteomyelitis demonstrated 12.1% of patients in each group with repeat wound recurrence, which could progress to new bone inoculation.[66] Therefore, proper eradication of soft tissue infection and resection of osteomyelitic bone and timely wound healing is paramount. Often partially ablative digital or ray pedal amputations are necessary to reduce risk of recurrence. Some newer studies have found no major dehiscence or ulcer recurrence when osteomyelitic bone was internally resected in 206 patients with diabetes, avoiding minor foot amputations.[67] In 2012, a study of 81 patients with diabetes and osteomyelitis demonstrated an overall limb salvage rate of 98.8%, with only a 16.9% recurrence of osteomyelitis.[68] Almost 25% of the patients required repeat operations for persistent infection, further solidifying the importance of eradication of all soft tissue and bone infection before hospital discharge.[68]

Although it is extremely difficult to obtain further understanding of the true recurrence of osteomyelitis in previously treated DFI, a standard method of outcomes and data collection and reporting would have to be followed. For example, after clinical and surgical cure of the current infection, each patient would have to be closely monitored for the duration and route of antibiotics given, presence of bacteria before definitive wound closure, usage of antibiotic-impregnated delivery systems, postoperative wound care, and length of follow-up. These are just a few of the parameters that would need to be consistent between reporting authors to gain a better understanding of recurrence rates. As the burden of cost related to health care dollars continues to come under scrutiny, more research will continue to be published looking at different way to prevent cost related to treatment of patients with diabetes, a large portion of allocated funding.

SUMMARY

The patient with diabetes with soft tissue and bone infection continues to challenge the treating surgeon. However, the published data available are expanding and providing new means of addressing these tough cases. The diagnosis and degree of infection should be made in a timely manner to determine if surgical intervention is also warranted. A strict, patient-focused protocol should then be followed for antibiotic selection, preoperative optimization and revascularization if necessary, surgical approach and debridement with consideration for antibiotic-impregnated implants, definitive wound closure, and postoperative follow-up. Ultimately, a multidisciplinary medical and surgical approach to the patient with DFI provides a more reproducible outcome, allowing for preservation of limb function and ambulation.

REFERENCES

1. Richard JL, Lavigne JP, Sotto A. Diabetes and foot infection: more than double trouble. Diabetes Metab Res Rev 2012;28(Suppl 1):46–53.
2. Bakker K, Schaper NC. The development of global consensus guidelines on the management and prevention of the diabetic foot 2011. Diabetes Metab Res Rev 2012;28(Suppl 1):116–8.
3. Lipsky BA, Berendt AR, Cornia PB, et al. 2012 Infectious Diseases Society of America Clinical Practice Guideline for the diagnosis and treatment of diabetic foot infections. Clin Infect Dis 2012;54(12):132–73.
4. Lipsky BA, Peters EJ, Senneville E, et al. Expert opinion on the management of infections in the diabetic foot. Diabetes Metab Res Rev 2012;28(Suppl 1):163–78.
5. Gardner SE, Hillis SL, Frantz RA. Clinical signs of infection in diabetic foot ulcers with high microbial load. Biol Res Nurs 2009;11(2):119–28.
6. Berendt AR, Peters EJ, Bakker K, et al. Diabetic foot osteomyelitis: a progress report on diagnosis and a systematic review of treatment. Diabetes Metab Res Rev 2008;24(Suppl 1):S145–61.
7. Grayson ML, Gibbons GW, Balogh K, et al. Probing to bone in infected pedal ulcers: a clinical sign of underlying osteomyelitis in diabetic patients. JAMA 1995;273:721.
8. Shone A, Burnside J, Chipchase S, et al. Probing the validity of the probe-to-bone test in the diagnosis of osteomyelitis of the foot in diabetes [letter]. Diabetes Care 2006;29:945.
9. Lavery LA, Armstrong DG, Peters EJ, et al. Probe-to-bone test for diagnosing diabetic foot osteomyelitis: reliable or relic? Diabetes Care 2007;30:270.
10. Mutluoglu M, Uzun G, Sildiroglu O, et al. Performance of the probe-to-bone test in a population suspected of having osteomyelitis of the foot in diabetes. JAMA 2012;102(5):369–73.
11. Jeffcoate WJ, Lipsky BA. Controversies in diagnosing and managing osteomyelitis of the foot in diabetes. Clin Infect Dis 2004;39(Suppl 2):S115.
12. Palestro CJ, Love C. Nuclear medicine and diabetic foot infections. Semin Nucl Med 2009;39(1):52–65.
13. Nawaz A, Torigian DA, Siegelman ES, et al. Diagnostic performance of FDG-PET, MRI, and plain film radiography (PFR) for the diagnosis of osteomyelitis in the diabetic foot. Mol Imaging Biol 2010;12(3):335–42.
14. Meyr AJ, Singh S, Zhang X. Statistical reliability of bone biopsy for the diagnosis of diabetic foot osteomyelitis. J Foot Ankle Surg 2011;50(6):663–7. http://dx.doi.org/10.1053/j.jfas.2011.08.005. Epub 2011 Sep 9. PMID:21907594.
15. Lipsky BA. Bone of contention: diagnosing the diabetic foot osteomyelitis. Clin Infect Dis 2008;47(4):528–30.
16. Frykberg RG. Team approach toward lower extremity amputation prevention in diabetes. J Am Podiatr Med Assoc 1997;87:305–12.
17. Sumpio BE, Aruny J, Blume PA. The multidisciplinary approach to limb salvage. Acta Chir Belg 2004;104:647–53.
18. Goldman FG. Deep space infections in the diabetic patients. J Am Podiatr Med Assoc 1987;77:431–43.
19. Van Baal JG. Surgical treatment of the infected diabetic foot. Clin Infect Dis 2004;39(Suppl 2):S123–8.

20. Lee BY, Guerra VJ, Civelek B. Compartment syndrome in the diabetic foot. Adv Wound Care 1995;3:36–46.
21. Rauwerda JA. Foot debridement: anatomic knowledge is mandatory. Diabetes Metab Res Rev 2000;16(Suppl 1):S23–6.
22. Aragon-Sanchez J, Lazaro-Martinez JL, Pulido-Duque J, et al. From the diabetic foot ulcer and beyond: how do foot infections spread in patients with diabetes? Diabet Foot Ankle 2012. http://dx.doi.org/10.3402/dfa.v3i0.18693.
23. Taylor GI, Minabe T. The angiosomes of mammals and other vertebrates. Plast Reconstr Surg 1992;89(2):181–215.
24. Taylor GI, Pan WR. Angiosomes of the leg: anatomic study and clinical implications. Plast Reconstr Surg 1998;102(3):599–616.
25. Attinger CE, Evans KK, Bulan E, et al. Angiosomes of the foot and ankle and clinical implications for limb salvage: reconstruction, incisions, and revascularization. Plast Reconstr Surg 2006;117(Suppl 7):S261–93.
26. Menzoian JO, LaMorte WW, Paniszyn CC, et al. Symptomatology and anatomic patterns of peripheral vascular disease: differing impact of smoking and diabetes. Ann Vasc Surg 1989;3:224–8.
27. Hobizal KB, Wukich DK. Diabetic foot infections: current concepts review. Diabet Foot Ankle 2012. http://dx.doi.org/10.3402/dfa.v3i0.18754.
28. Chakraborti C, Le C, Yanofsky A. Sensitivity of superficial cultures in lower extremity wounds. J Hosp Med 2010;5:415–20.
29. Lipsky BA. Osteomyelitis of the foot in diabetic patients. Clin Infect Dis 1997;25: 1318–26.
30. Lipsky BA. A report from the international consensus on diagnosing and treating the infected diabetic foot. Diabetes Metab Res Rev 2004;20:568–77.
31. Levin LS. The reconstructive ladder. An orthoplastic approach. Orthop Clin North Am 1993;24(3):393–409.
32. Gottlieb LJ, Krieger LM. From the reconstructive ladder to the reconstructive elevator. Plast Reconstr Surg 1994;93(7):1503–4.
33. Janis JE, Kwon RK, Attinger CE. The new reconstructive ladder. Modifications to the traditional model. Plast Reconstr Surg 2011;127:205S–12S.
34. Capobianco CM, Stapleton JJ, Zgonis T. Soft tissue reconstruction pyramid in the diabetic foot. Foot Ankle Spec 2010;3(5):241–8.
35. Zgonis T, Stapleton JJ, Roukis TS. Advanced plastic surgery techniques for soft tissue coverage of the diabetic foot. Clin Podiatr Med Surg 2007;24(3): 547–68.
36. Pinzur MA, Sage R, Abraham M, et al. Limb salvage in infected lower extremity gangrene. Foot Ankle 1988;8(4):212–5.
37. Scher KS, Steele FJ. The septic foot in patients with diabetes. Surgery 1988; 104(4):661–6.
38. Donato MC, Novicki DC, Blume PA. Skin grafting: historic and practical approaches. Clin Podiatr Med Surg 2000;17(4):561–98.
39. Roukis TS, Zgonis T. Skin grafting techniques for soft-tissue coverage of diabetic foot and ankle wounds. J Wound Care 2005;14(4):173–6.
40. Llanos S, Danilla S, Barraza C, et al. Effectiveness of negative-pressure closure in the integration of split thickness skin grafts: a randomized, double-masked, controlled trial. Ann Surg 2006;244(5):700–5.
41. Nakayama Y, Iino T, Soeda S. A new method for the dressing of free skin grafts. Plast Reconstr Surg 1990;86(6):1216–9.
42. Attinger CE, Ducic I, Zelen C. The use of local muscle flaps in foot and ankle reconstruction. Clin Podiatr Med Surg 2000;17(4):681–711.

43. Attinger CE, Ducic I, Cooper P, et al. The role of intrinsic muscle flaps of the foot for bone coverage in foot and ankle defects in diabetic and nondiabetic patients. Plast Reconstr Surg 2002;110(4):1047–54.

44. Baumeister SP, Spierer R, Erdmann D, et al. A realistic complication analysis of 70 sural artery flaps in a multimorbid patient group. Plast Reconstr Surg 2003; 112(1):129–40.

45. Noack N, Hartmann B, Kuntscher MV. Measures to prevent complications of distally based neurovascular sural flaps. Ann Plast Surg 2006;57(1):37–40.

46. Tosun Z, Ozkan A, Karacor Z, et al. Delaying the reverse sural flap provides predictable results for complicated wounds in diabetic foot. Ann Plast Surg 2005;54(5):562–5.

47. Buchholz H, Engelbrecht H. Uber die depotwirkung eineger antibiotica bei vermischung mit dem kunstharz palacos. Chirurg 1970;41(11):511–5.

48. Roeder B, Van Gils CC, Maling S. Antibiotic beads in the treatment of diabetic pedal osteomyelitis. J Foot Ankle Surg 2000;39(2):124–30.

49. Klemm K. Antibiotic bead chains. Clin Orthop 1993;(295):63–76.

50. Fish D, Hoffman H, Danzinger L. Antibiotic-impregnated cement use in U.S. hospitals. Am J Hosp Pharm 1992;49:2469–74.

51. Nelson CL, Hiddman SG, Harrison BH. Orthopedic infections: elution characteristics of gentamicin-PMMA beads after implantation in humans. Orthopedics 1994;17(5):415–6.

52. Henry SI, Hood GA, Seligson D. Long-term implantation of gentamicin-polymethylmethacrylate antibiotic beads. Clin Orthop Relat Res 1993;(295):47–53.

53. Hanssen AD. Local antibiotic delivery vehicles in the treatment of musculoskeletal infection. Clin Orthop Relat Res 2005;(437):91–6.

54. DeSilva GL, Fritzler A, DeSilva SP. Antibiotic-impregnated cement spacer for bone defects of the forearm and hand. Tech Hand Up Extrem Surg 2007; 11(2):163–7.

55. Schade VL, Roukis TS. The role of polymethylmethacrylate antibiotic-loaded cement in addition to debridement for the treatment of soft tissue and osseous infections of the foot and ankle. J Foot Ankle Surg 2010;49:55–62.

56. Calhoun JH, Klemm K, Anger DM, et al. Use of antibiotic-PMMA beads in the ischemic foot. Orthopedics 1994;17(5):453–7.

57. Fabian GK, deVries G, Meakin C, et al. Outcome of transmetatarsal amputations in diabetes using antibiotic beads. Foot Ankle Int 2009;30(6):486–93.

58. Vardakas KZ, Horianopoulou M, Falagas ME. Factors associated with treatment failure in patients with diabetic foot infections: an analysis of data from randomized controlled trials. Diabetes Res Clin Pract 2008;80:344–51.

59. Pittet D, Wyssa B, Herter-Clavel C, et al. Outcome of diabetic foot infections treated conservatively: a retrospective cohort study with long-term follow-up. Arch Intern Med 1999;159:851–6.

60. Mutluoglu M, Sivrioglu AK, Eroglu M, et al. The implications of the presence of osteomyelitis on outcomes of infected diabetic foot wounds. Scand J Infect Dis 2013;45(7):497–503.

61. Oh TS, Lee HS, Hong JP. Diabetic foot reconstruction using free flaps increases 5-year-survival rate. J Plast Reconstr Aesthet Surg 2013;66(2):243–50.

62. Kadukammakal J, Yau S, Urbas W. Assessment of partial first-ray resections and their tendency to progress to transmetatarsal amputations: a retrospective study. J Am Podiatr Med Assoc 2012;102(5):412–6.

63. National diabetes fact sheet, 2011. Atlanta (GA): US Department of Health and Human Services. Center for Disease Control and Prevention; 2011.

64. Borkosky SL, Roukis TS. Incidence of re-amputation following partial first ray amputation associated with diabetes mellitus and peripheral sensory neuropathy: a systematic review. Diabet Foot Ankle 2012. http://dx.doi.org/10.3402/dfa.v3i0.12169.

65. Pascale R, Vitale M, Esposito S, et al. Update on diabetic foot infections. Infez Med 2012;20(3):155–68.

66. Widatalla AH, Mahadi SE, Shawer MA, et al. Diabetic foot infections with osteomyelitis: efficacy of combined surgical and medical treatment. Diabet Foot Ankle 2012. http://dx.doi.org/10.3402/dfa.v3i0.18809.

67. Faglia E, Clerici G, Caminiti M, et al. Feasibility and effectiveness of internal pedal amputation of phalanx or metatarsal head in diabetic patients with forefoot osteomyelitis. J Foot Ankle Surg 2012;51(5):593–8.

68. Aragon-Sanchez J, Lazaro-Martinez JL, Hernandez-Herrero C, et al. Does osteomyelitis in the feet of patients with diabetes really recur after surgical treatment? Natural history of a surgical series. Diabet Med 2012;29(6):813–8.

Offloading of the Diabetic Foot
Orthotic and Pedorthic Strategies

Brant L. McCartan, DPM, MBA, MS[a,b,]*, Barry I. Rosenblum, DPM[a]

KEYWORDS

- Orthoses • Diabetes • Ulceration • Offloading • Bracing • Monitoring
- Team approach • Modifications

KEY POINTS

- Each foot must be treated independently. What works for one side may not be successful for the contralateral limb in the same patient or in other similar patients.
- The balance between what is functional and that which accommodates is a challenge for the entire team. Currently, the most appropriate materials are short lasting and must be replaced routinely.
- The diabetic foot constantly changes with time, body habitus, and systemic conditions— patients and their care takers must be educated to watch for warning signs and seek early intervention.
- Follow-up for regular monitoring, maintenance, and modifications of orthotic and pedorthic devices is crucial for successful prevention of further collapse or reulceration.
- In even the most compliant patients wearing the best devices, devices breakdown at times. The importance of always wearing a device cannot be overemphasized. Patients need to be able to apply a brace and function with the orthoses - they need to want to wear them.

INTRODUCTION: NATURE OF THE PROBLEM

The diabetic foot, at times, is an anomaly to even the most seasoned practitioners. Decreased circulation and sensation leave the limb almost destined to ulceration, collapse, or often both. Once this occurs, the susceptibility to infection and amputation is heightened. The principles of ulcer treatment have remained constant despite the technological advances of medicines, dressings, and biologic skin equivalents.

[a] Beth Israel Deaconess Medical Center, Harvard Medical School, 185 Pilgrim Road, Baker Span 3, Boston, MA 02215, USA; [b] Private Practice, Milwaukee Foot Specialists, 3610 Michelle Witmer Memorial Drive, Suite 110, New Berlin, WI 53151, USA
* Corresponding author. Milwaukee Foot Specialists, 3610 Michelle Witmer Memorial Drive, Suite 110, New Berlin, WI 53151, USA.
E-mail address: dr.mccartan@yahoo.com

Clin Podiatr Med Surg 31 (2014) 71–88
http://dx.doi.org/10.1016/j.cpm.2013.09.004
0891-8422/14/$ – see front matter © 2014 Elsevier Inc. All rights reserved.

Keys to ulcer treatment
- Infection control
- Maximizing perfusion
- Adequate nutrition
- Offloading

Offloading of the diabetic foot entails a lifetime of work and encompasses the time from initial presentation to perioperative period to postoperative management. The foot structure is in a contact flux; fluid management of patients can lead to rapid weight gains and loses. Limb swelling and neuropathy make education of patients and their caretakers paramount because regular modifications are necessary. These can be performed by a multitude of health professionals, but the best management is a team approach with regular follow-up and a watchful eye.

THERAPEUTIC OPTIONS

Orthoses and braces can be used for every type of patient. These devices are used in diabetic patients to prevent ulceration or reulceration and serve to brace or accommodate a collapsing or collapsed foot. They reduce peak plantar pressures in the foot.[1–3] There are 2 specific types of orthoses, functional and accommodative. Typically rigid orthoses are thought to best functionally correct a flexible, biomechanical abnormality. Soft orthoses accommodate a misshapen or painful rigid foot. In diabetic patients, the extremes must be avoided. There is a balance between accommodating a misshapen foot structure and helping to function as a brace to prevent further collapse. The concept of total contact, no matter if an orthotic or cast is used, helps disperse pressure evenly off of prominent areas and helps maintain current joint architecture.

Diabetic patients are at an increased risk during the intraoperative period compared with nondiabetic patients. Orthoses and bracing can help prevent surgery. Sometimes, however, surgery is unavoidable. Luckily, different devices can prolong the time to surgery. They can also serve as an intermediary in the perioperative period to help close an ulceration before an exostectomy or reconstruction. They also can be used postoperatively to bridge a patient between a cast and their normal shoe gear.

DIFFERENT INITIAL PRESENTATIONS
Ideal Foot

The diabetic foot can present in a multitude of conditions. The ideal presentation is to see a foot that has not collapsed or ulcerated in a well-educated, well-controlled patient. **Table 1** depicts a good algorithm for patients who have intact neurovascular status and are compliant with a normal-appearing foot. Certainly most standard shoes are acceptable. If a patient is neuropathic, it is beneficial to offer an extra depth shoe (**Fig. 1**) or, if hammertoes are present, a shoe with an elastic toe box (**Fig. 2**)

Table 1 Algorithm to treating an "Ideal" diabetic foot – one without collapse or calluses, in a patient with neuropathy, or increased susceptibility to deformity, collapse or ulceration				
Condition of Foot	Shoes	Orthoses	Braces	Follow-up
"Ideal"	Correct fit	± for Comfort	None	Annual CDFE Education of warning signs
Ischemic/neuropathic	Extra depth	Accommodative	None	More frequent follow-up

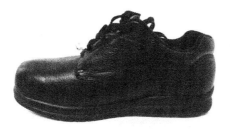

Fig. 1. Extra depth shoe – note increased height of toe box.

that stretches to accommodate the toes is helpful. An annual comprehensive diabetic foot examination (CDFE) is a good screening to help catch abnormalities before they become worse.

Diabetic Foot with Preulcerative Callus

In patients with a preulcerative callus (**Fig. 3**), the cause must be determined. Is it strictly from increased plantar pressure or too tight shoe gear? Is there increased shearing from a biomechanical abnormality? **Table 2** demonstrates a variety of scenarios. Ulcers frequently result from areas of callus.[4] The shear forces cause microseparation between skin layers and cause damage to the tissues deeper to the epidermis.[5] Routine débridements of the thickened, hypertrophic tissue help decrease pressure to the area.

Diabetic Foot with Ulceration

If a patient presents with an ulceration, it must be managed. The infection must be controlled and vascular status assessed and optimized. Depth should be analyzed, especially which tissue plane is exposed: through dermis, muscle, capsule, and

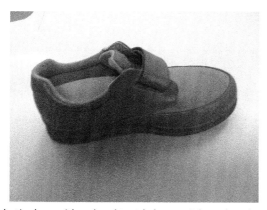

Fig. 2. Custom diabetic shoe with nylon (stretchy) material on dorsal aspect of toe box to allow room for rigid hammertoes or distal bony prominences.

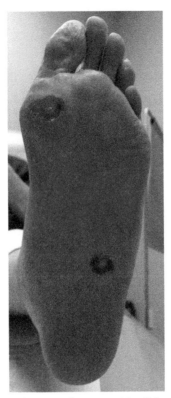

Fig. 3. Pre-ulcerative calluses on bottom of neuropathic, diabetic foot representing areas of increased pressure.

bone. Once the emergent factors are addressed, pressure reduction is the most controllable therapy for successful salvage. Again, the biomechanical cause of the ulceration must be determined. **Fig. 4** depicts a patient with a lateral foot ulceration. This ulceration results from a decreased eversion strength, leaving the foot in a varus

Table 2
Algorithm to treat diabetic patients with a pre-ulcerative callus depending on cause and location

Condition of Foot	Shoes	Orthoses	Braces	Follow-up
Dorsal calluses over IPJs	Extra depth with flexible doral toe box	± for Control	None	Regular
Medial pinch callus or styloid	Correct fit	Functional	None	Regular
Plantar forefoot or midfoot	Extra depth	Accommodative, and modified to offload prominent areas of greatest peak plantar pressure	None	Quarterly
Flexible flatfoot (posterior tibial tendon dysfunction)	Comfort or extra depth	Built into brace	Guantlet	Annual

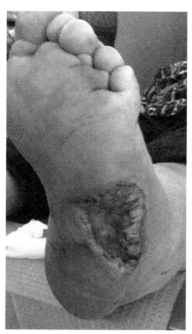

Fig. 4. Ulcer along lateral column. Note equinovarus contracture and position of foot due to lateral muscle weakness and subsequent decrease eversion strength.

attitude. Wounds like this are challenging to treat, but they are even more difficult to prevent from coming back. Bracing is a must if surgical correction is not possible. Ulceration is the precursor to amputation for most diabetic patients.[6–9] Total contact casting (TCC) remains the gold standard for ulceration offloading. TCCs are especially useful for plantar midfoot ulcerations or in patients with active Charcot joint collapse. In addition, if a patient has muscle weakness causing a deformity, such as drop foot, bracing is required. The shoes must also be able to house the brace (**Table 3**).

Table 3
Algorithm to treat diabetic patients with more severe deformities, collapse or ulcerations at specific regions of the foot

Condition of Foot	Shoes	Orthoses	Braces	Follow-up
Dorsal ulceration	Extra depth	± for Control	None	Weekly until healed
Plantar ulceration	Extra depth once healed	Accommodative and modified to offload ulcer. May need to consider regular dressing changes	TCC, felted-foam	Weekly or more frequent
Plantar cuboid, Charcot	N/A	Plastizote built into brace	CROW	
Dropfoot	Extra depth to accommodate brace	Accommodative to disperse pressure	AFO	Regular

Diabetic Foot Requiring Surgical Correction

At times, surgery is required. In the preoperative period, orthoses can be used to offload and help reduce the ulcer size or, ideally, heal the ulceration. **Table 4** represents a variety of challenging scenarios. After this, definitive surgery can be performed. Patients with equinus as the culprit of increased forefoot pressure often require soft tissue release (tendo-Achilles lengthening, gastrocneumius recession, or targeted plantar fascia release). Boots and casts are used to maintain the correction in the perioperative period. Postoperatively, the foot adapts. Similarly to how a residual limb changes and molds for a prosthetic, the foot accommodates. Areas that were not prominent before may become the most prominent area after exostectomy.

During reconstruction and creation of an arch, there may be new areas that become more susceptible to injury and need to be addressed. During the longer-term postoperative period, adventitious bursa or bursitis can form. The bursa should diminish in size with proper offloading. If it becomes too large, it can cause reulceration and may need to be excised. The bony prominence deep to the bursa may require additional resection. During reconstructions, hardware is often placed and prevention of an ulcer (portal of entry for bacteria) is vital. As the foot changes and accommodates, so must the orthotic devices. Braces can be used to correct flexible deformities, muscle weaknesses, and wasting due to neuropathy. Many times, a normal-appearing foot is not achievable during surgery, and efforts are directed to create a foot that is functional only with a brace. **Fig. 5** is a picture of a patient's shoe and brace modification after a partial calcanectomy. Extra effort must be paid not only to supporting this patient's ankle but also directed at prevented a plantar calcaneal ulceration. Postoperatively, an amputation or fusion changes a patient's gait; bracing is required. Shoe filler helps further stabilize the foot in the shoe after single digit or multiple forefoot amputations (**Fig. 6**). Patients typically prefer wearing shoes with similar appearance. With more proximal amputations, however, this is not always possible, and a short shoe has to suffice (**Fig. 7**). Different

Table 4
Algorithm to treat or temporize diabetic patients requiring surgical intervention and methods to stabilize feet post-operatively to prevent subsequent surgeries

Condition of Foot	Shoes	Orthoses	Braces	Follow-up
Immediate postoperative	Postoperative shoe	None	Short leg cast Posterior splint Removable walking cast	Weekly or more frequent
Healed incision	Extra depth	Accommodative	Gauntlet, AFO, CROW	Very regular with multiple health professionals when applying new shoes or braces
Postamputation	Extra depth	Accommodative with shoe filler	± Based on need	Regular adjustments
Unrepairable, not a surgical candidate, failed surgery	Extra depth	Built into brace	Patellar-tendon device	Regular adjustments

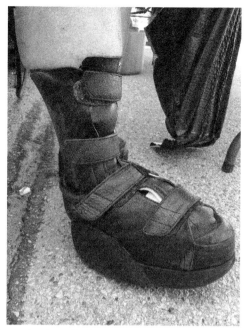

Fig. 5. Foot with calcaneal gait and subsequent partial calcanectomy. Note combination of proximal brace and rocker shoe to help off-load high pressure areas.

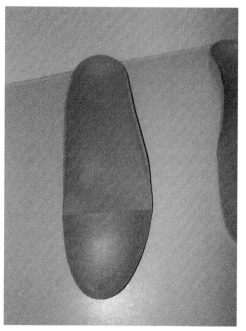

Fig. 6. Plastizote accommodative orthotic with toe filler to help stabilize foot by filling the void status post amputation.

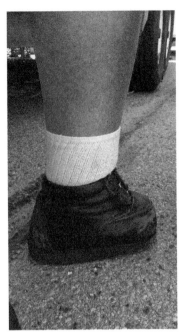

Fig. 7. Short shoe for patient status post proximal amputation.

amputation levels also result in alteration of biomechanics. Bracing can be used to restore a lever arm lost from a digital or transmetatarsal amputation.[10,11] Some patients require an ankle-foot orthosis (AFO) to compensate for the loss of lever arm or flexion strength (**Fig. 8**).

CLINICAL CORRELATION AND OUTCOMES

Improper shoe fitting can cause skin breakdown. High plantar pressure and shear force is another factor. These can be curbed by foot orthoses and bracing. If a brace does not fit properly, however, ulceration may ensue. Shoe and brace selection must be geared at making it easy for patients to maintain compliance and be easy to apply with a pleasant appearance. This becomes more difficult as the demands of and on the device increase. The devices must be modifiable as the foot changes, and they must be able to accommodate a brace.

Orthotic Materials

Orthotic materials, in general, must offload the current deformity and prevent future breakdown. This is best accomplished by dispersing plantar forces and stabilizing the foot to prevent shearing. Attention should be directed at restoring gait. If the deformities are reducible and flexible, bracing is a great conservative option. It is best to have a multilayered device. The base layer should be the most dense, and density or durometer should decrease up the device toward contact with the foot. Ethylene vinyl acetate (EVA) and 60-mm Poron are stable and easy to work with. It is the material of choice to balance out a deformity and is a good base layer. Plastizote is a great top layer or in direct contact with the foot (**Fig. 9**). It comes in varying densities and is modifiable but does break down more rapidly than cork and other materials. Some

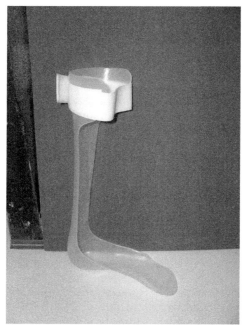

Fig. 8. Rigid ankle-foot orthoses to help keep patients ankle in a more rectus position. Used for patients with weakened extensor strength and multiplanar deformities.

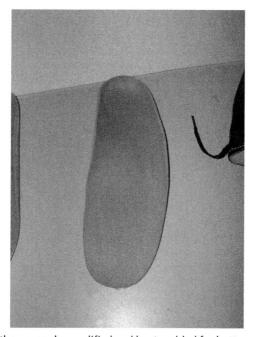

Fig. 9. Plastizote orthoses, can be modified and heat molded for better accommodation and off-loading. Typically breaks down after four months, but great at reducing pressure.

studies support a 3-layer orthotic consisting of a moldable polyethylene foam in contact with the foot, a middle urethane polymer layer for shock absorption, and a firm cork or EVA base layer for functional support and control.[12,13] Extra depth shoes are best with patients having rigid hammertoes or requiring a brace, such as an AFO.[14]

Therapeutic Shoes

Therapeutic shoes are traditionally extra depth (increased by at least one-quarter inch) and rocker soled. One study determined that "comfort shoes" are better than extra depth without an orthotic at reducing forefoot pressure.[1] Extra depth shoes with an orthotic were found, however, to greater reduce pressure, especially with a rocker bottom. If possible, the shoe should be made of breathable materials, such as leather or Gore-Tex. Slip-on shoes are easy to put on but lack stability and are often too tight once the foot slips forward. In addition, they do not hold braces or orthoses well.

Rocker Bottom

Rocker bottom shoes help offload plantar pressure in the forefoot, but are dependent on the placement of the rocker. This is particularly important because many diabetic ulcers occur in the forefoot.[15,16] Rockers help transition the foot from heel strike to toe-off. This restores normal motion as a result of collapse, stiffness, and fusion and improves the gait. Praet and Louwerens[17] discuss the rocker is the best way to offload the forefoot. The positioning of the apex of the rocker is most important. This must be custom for diabetics suffering from calluses or ulcers in specific areas or with foot collapse. Similar to a metatarsal pad, the best placement of the apex is just proximal to the area where pressure relief is desired. If there is a plantar metatarsal ulceration, the apex should be right at the neck of the metatarsals to offload the metatarsal head(s) involved. There are a handful of different rocker bottom designs.[14,18] The basic concept is just that of a rocking chair. A mild midstance (where the shoe contacts the ground) is most common and helps restore gait. Depending on severity of deformity and stiffness of joints, this can be altered and increased. It is also easy to incorporate a lift to even out a limb length discrepancy (**Fig. 10**). An example where a more severe rocker is required is a patient who has both submetatarsal head ulcerations and distal toe tip ulcerations. In patients with decreased sensation or inability to achieve toe-off, a rigid shank may be useful. This adds weight but decreases motion at the midfoot and

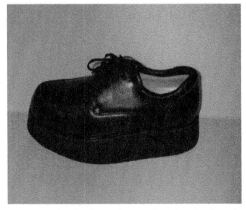

Fig. 10. Rocker bottom, extra-depth shoe. Apex of rocker is placed proximally to desired area to off-load. In this example just proximal to the metatarsal heads.

forefoot. In addition to orthoses and shoes, wearing two sets of socks can be helpful—this allows some of the shearing to take place between the two layers and decreases the movement between the skin and sock interface.

The deformity must be captured to reduce the greatest amount of plantar pressure. Scanners are easy to use; however, there is equal success with traditional casting or foam block methods. It may be easiest for patients to swing their legs over and get an impression with the foam box at a semi–weight-bearing position. As seen in (**Fig. 11**), the calluses can be marked to help the orthotic company visualize areas of pressure. Further offloading can be created when using the foam box as well (**Fig. 12**). The hips, legs, and ankle should be at right angles, and, once the subtalar joint is in neutral (assuming flexibility), even pressure must be applied to capture the contour of the foot (**Fig. 13**).[2] Again, using a modifiable material to create the orthoses is important because changes in the foot can occur even between the times of casting and application. Customization is key with multiple levels of amputation.

Braces

The proper use of a brace is important to offload the diabetic foot, whether in the acute phase, such as seen with an ulceration or Charcot deformity, or in the chronic stages, when healing is taking place and prevention is the primary goal of therapy. In this discussion, bracing techniques are any product that extends above the level of the malleoli.

For flexible deformities, a semirigid gauntlet type of device may suffice. Braces are able to restrict motion, so if there is some instability brought on my motor weakness or loss of function, this may be the ideal solution. Patients with a combination of sensory neuropathy and a collapsing medial column, whether from Charcot neuroarthropathy or posterior tibial tendon dysfunction, may benefit from a gauntlet device (**Fig. 14**).

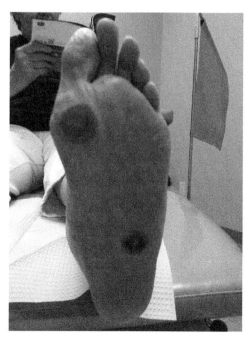

Fig. 11. Example of ways to indicate areas of greatest pressure and prominence – mark foot directly before casting.

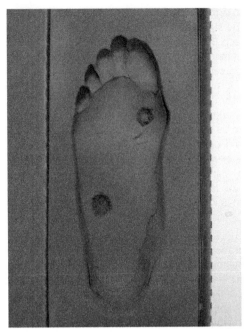

Fig. 12. Example of markings on foam-box of areas of greatest pressure to off-load in orthoses.

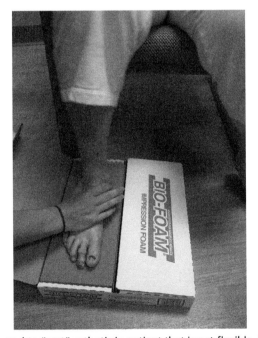

Fig. 13. Technique used to "cast" orthotic in patient that is not flexible. Notice knee is bent at 90 degrees as well as ankle. Attention directed at putting patient in subtalar joint neutral.

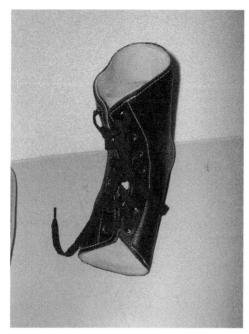

Fig. 14. Gauntlet device used for patients with ankle and or subtalar joint arthritis, Posterior Tibial Tendon dysfunction, or more severe collapse. Helps to stabilize deformity and decrease motion.

Ankle-foot Orthosis

AFO is indicated (**Fig. 15**) for more rigid deformities. Care must be taken in the neuropathic foot to avoid any areas that may be irritated or lead to additional problems. Complications may arise from any of these devices discussed, including the AFO, which, of all the braces discussed, is likely the most cost effective. For those patients with motor weakness, it helps to accommodate weakness in dorsiflexion and may also be used, along with the possibility of the gauntlet, for those who have had a partial foot amputation and have a frontal plane deformity, either in inversion or eversion.

Charcot Restraint Orthotic Walker

Charcot restraint orthotic walkers (CROWs) are often required for those patients with severe deformities or Charcot in its acute phase (**Fig. 16**). This device is custom made and is essentially a clamshell device made out of polypropylene. It is designed for the long term but is not meant to be permanent. The CROW may also be used for patients with Charcot and an active ulcer. Lastly, the CROW may be used after a Charcot reconstruction.

Total Contact Cast

Total contact cast (TCC) must be discussed, because a discussion of bracing of the foot is not complete without its mention. The standard of care is always being challenged with technology. The TCC, however, remains the gold standard for offloading.[19] An often-quoted meta analysis[20] shows the average time to heal an ulceration decreased 184 days to 44 days with the use of a TCC.[12,21,22] Possibly the greatest advantage of these is that patients cannot take them off. Some studies

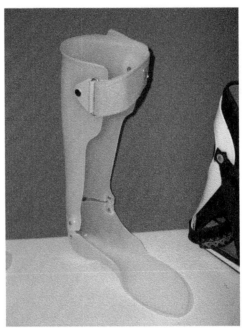

Fig. 15. Hinged ankle-foot orthotic used for patients that require some ankle motion.

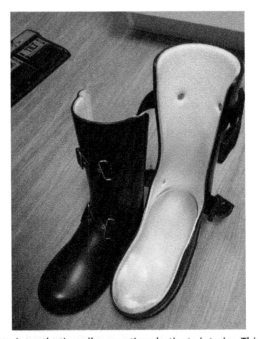

Fig. 16. Charcot restraint orthotic walker – notice plastizote interior. This clam shell appearing device is used for an unstable ankle, rearfoot and midfoot by dispersing pressures up the leg. Lower durometer plastizote is used on the plantar surface to further reduce pressure and accommodate deformity.

have shown that patients offloaded with removable cast boots walked without them 72% of the time.[12] For midfoot ulcerations where offloading is a challenge, TCCs work well. Despite all the positive evidence, a study of 895 wound care clinics in the United States showed less than 2% of clinicians use a TCC to offload a diabetic wound.[23] In the clinical setting with less challenging wounds or wounds that require daily dressing changes, felted-foam dressings can be of benefit.[24] These have less restriction, allow for dressing changes, can be applied quickly in the office, and can bridge patients while they are waiting for custom orthoses. Unfortunately, not all patients can accommodate a brace within their shoe and require an external device attached to the shoe (**Fig. 17**). This may be more cumbersome—but it allows patients to ambulate safely. A team approach using an orthotist and pedorthist is crucial because constant modifications are required—customization is the key (**Fig. 18**).

Finally, for those patients who are either not candidates for reconstruction or who have had reconstructions that have failed, it may be necessary to offload the limb more proximally. This may be accomplished with a patellar-tendon type of device (**Fig. 19**). Although essentially creating the same mechanics as a prosthetic limb, this device serves to redistribute pressure and weight-bearing forces more proximal to, as the name suggests, the prepatella area. There are many ways that this may be fabricated.

COMPLICATIONS AND CONCERNS

The clinical outcome of using orthoses or preventing reulceration status postsurgery is determined by the vigilance of patients and treating teams. As discussed in this article,

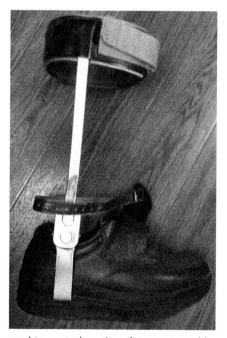

Fig. 17. External device used to control motion about an unstable ankle. Used for patients that cannot be accommodated with an internal device due to severity of deformity.

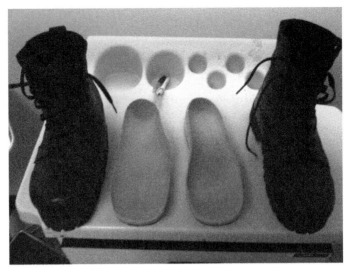

Fig. 18. Example of some of the tools required to modify devices in-office.

constant attention must be paid to hot spots and more prominent areas to prevent ulceration. Braces can cause discomfort and, if bulky in appearance, many patients refuse to wear them. They can also create new ulcerations. The highest risk factor for developing an ulceration is the history of a previous ulcer.[25,26] The highest risk times once treatment has begun are when new shoes, orthoses, or braces are used.[27,28] Time to follow-up should be short on application of new footgear. Do not

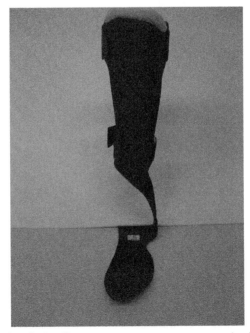

Fig. 19. Patellar-tendon device disperses pressures even more proximally up the leg.

dispense a device and discharge a patient. This is the most crucial time to prevent further breakdown.

Tips to avoid complications
- When dispensing new orthoses or braces, regular follow-up in the initial weeks to month helps quickly find and correct hot spots, or areas of unwanted pressure.
- If dispensing diabetic shoes with multiple pairs of orthoses, give patients a sticker or a reminder to put on their calendar to change orthoses every 3 to 4 months. Also, if patients are seen regularly for routine care, time their appointments around when it is right to switch out their orthoses.
- If the foot architecture is supported correctly by custom shoes, orthoses, and braces, there is less work for the lower extremity muscles and ligaments. As these structures adapt and the hypertrophied muscles return to normal size, modifications are required to maintain a good fit. Quarterly or semiannual maintenance is a good idea the first year or if patients have an increase in weight loss or weight gain.
- Do not leave patients stranded while waiting for their custom devices. Temporary support should be fabricated until the permanent shoe, orthotic, or brace is ready.
- When an ulceration is successfully closed, the new skin is not, and never will be, as strong as in its preulcerative state. Continue offloading this area until the skin strengthens and custom orthoses are ready.

SUMMARY

The diabetic foot frequently has bony prominences. These can be offloaded from the inside—surgical exostectomy or joint reconstruction—or from the outside—orthoses and bracing. Not every patient wants surgery or is even a candidate for surgery. With a well-trained team working together, orthoses can help prevent surgery as well as help avoid revisional surgery and postoperative breakdown. A recent study revealed that reulceration rate decreased from 79% to 15% 2 years after the initiation of orthotic therapy.[29] In this same study, amputation rate decreased from 54% to 6%. Education, reinforcement, and early intervention are paramount. Constant maintenance and modifications are required for lifelong success.

REFERENCES

1. Lavery LA, Vela SA, Fieischli JG, et al. Reducing plantar pressure in the neuropathic foot: a comparison of footwear. Diabetes Care 1997;20(11):1706–10.
2. Tsung BY, Zhang M, Mak AF, et al. Effectiveness of insoles on plantar pressure redistribution. J Rehabil Res Dev 2004;41(6A):767–74.
3. Viswanathan V, Madhavan S, Gopalakrishna G, et al. Effectiveness of different tyeps of footwear insoles for the diabetic neuropathic foot. Diabetes Care 2004; 27(2):474–7.
4. Murray HG, Young MJ, Hollis S, et al. The association between callus formation, high pressures and neuropathy in diabetic foot population. Diabet Med 1996;13: 979–82.
5. Sulzberger MB, Cortese TA, Fishman L, et al. Studies on blisters produced by friction. J Invest Dermatol 1966;47:456–65.
6. Reiber GE, Vileikyte L, Boyko EJ, et al. Causal pathways for incident lower extremity ulcers in patients with diabetes from two settings. Diabetes Care 1999; 22:157–62.
7. Sedory Holzer SE, Camerota A, Martens L, et al. Costs and durations of care for lower-extremity ulcers in patients with diabetes. Clin Ther 1998;20:169–81.

8. Ollendorf DA, Kotsanos JG, Wishner WJ, et al. Potential economic benefits of lower-extremity amputation prevention strategies in diabetes. Diabetes Care 1998;21:1240–5.

9. Slater R, Ramot Y, Rapoport M. Diabetic foot ulcers: principles of assessment and treatment. Isr Med Assoc J 2001;3:59–62.

10. Philbin TM, Leyes M, Sferra JJ, et al. Orthotic and prosthetic devices in partial foot amputations. Foot Ankle Clin 2001;6(2):215–28.

11. Rheinstein J, Yanke J, Marzano R. Developing an effective prescription for a lower extremity prosthesis. Foot Ankle Clin North Am 1999;4(1):113–39.

12. Janisse DJ. A scientific approach to insole design for the diabetic foot. Foot 1993; 3:105–8.

13. Janisse DJ. Pedorthic care of the diabetic foot. In: Levin ME, O'Neal LW, Bowker JR, editors. The diabetic foot. 5th edition. St Louis (MO): Mosby-Year Book; 1993. p. 549.

14. Janisse DJ. Prescription insoles and footwear. Clin Podiatr Med Surg 1995;1: 41–61.

15. Mueller MJ, Zou D, Lott DJ. Pressure gradient as an indicator of plantar skin injury. Diabetes Care 2005;28(12):2908–12.

16. Yavuz M, Erdermir A, Botek G, et al. Peak plantar pressure and shear locations. Diabetes Care 2007;30(10):2643–5.

17. Praet SF, Louwerens JK. The influence of shoe design on plantar pressures in neuropathic feet. Diabetes Care 2003;26:441–5.

18. Marzano R. Fabricating shoe modifications and foot orthoses. In: Janisse DJ, editor. Introduction to pedorthics. Columbia (MD): Pedorthic Footwear Association; 1998. p. 221–34.

19. Pollo FE, Brodsky JW, Crenshaw SJ, et al. Plantar pressures in fiberglass total contact casts vs. a new diabetic walking boot. FAI 2003;24(1):45–9.

20. Petre M, Tokar P, Kostar D, et al. Revisiting the total contact cast: maximizing off-loading by wound isolation. Diabetes Care 2005;28(4):929–30.

21. Brodsky JW, Kourosh S, Stills M, et al. Objective evaluation of insert material for diabetic and athletic footwear. Foot Ankle 1988;9:111.

22. Armstrong DG, Laveray LA, Kimbriel HR, et al. Activity patterns of patients with diabetic foot ulceration: patients with active ulceration may not adhere to a standard pressure off-loading regimen. Diabetes Care 2003;26(9):2595–7.

23. Wu SC, Jensen JL, Weber AK, et al. Use of pressure offloading devices in diabetic foot ulcers: do we practice what we preach? Diabetes Care 2008;31:2118.

24. Zimny S, Schatz H, Pfohl U. The effects of applied felted foam on wound healing and healing times in the therapy of neuropathic diabetic foot ulcers. Diabet Med 2003;20(8):622–5.

25. Edmonds ME, Blundell MP, Morris ME, et al. Improved survival of the diabetic foot: the role of a specialized foot clnic. Q J Med 1986;60(232):763–71.

26. Apelqvist J, Larsson J, Agardh CD. Long-term prognosis for diabetic patients with foot ulcers. J Intern Med 1993;233(6):485–91.

27. Apelqvist J, Larsson J, Agardh CD. The influence of external percipitatint factors and peripheral neuropathy on the development and outcome of diabetic foot ulcers. J Diabet Complications 1990;4(1):21–5.

28. Macarlane RM, Jeffcoate WJ. Factors contributing to the presentation of diabetic foot ulcers. Diabet Med 1997;14(10):867–70.

29. Fernandez ML, Lozano RM, Diaz MI. How effective is orthotic treatment in patients with recurrent diabetic foot ulcers? J Am Podiatr Med Assoc 2013; 103(4):281–90.

Bioengineered Alternative Tissues

Emily A. Cook, DPM, MPH*, Jeremy J. Cook, DPM, MPH,
Homan Badri, DPM, John Mostafa, DPM

KEYWORDS

- Diabetic • Bioengineered • skin • Acellular • Cellular • Ulcer

KEY POINTS

- Bioengineered alternative tissues(BATs) can be classified based on their cellular properties, derivations and structural composition. In our current review we simplified the classification of BATs into epidermal, dermal and bi-layer (epidermal/dermal) types.
- By presenting and fully understanding the evidence and approved indications for each type of BAT available on the market we can avoid the over utilization and misuse of BATs.
- It is crucial to understand the physiology and biological elements missing in the healing of chronic diabetic ulcers.
- Current BATs serve as protective barriers and are not geared for replacing skins higher complex functions.
- The holy grail of tissue replacement has yet to be discovered as skin stem cell regeneration research continues to overcome political debates.

Bioengineered alternative tissues (BATs) are a heterogeneous group of processed materials frequently used to aid in wound closure of diabetic foot ulcers (DFUs; Table 1). Kim and colleagues[1] first coined the term *bioengineered alternative tissue* in 2001. The impetus for finding a universal term was to eliminate the confusion of several names used in the worldwide literature. Despite the best efforts to unify all these ambiguous terms, the literature still uses different terms when describing the different types of BATs.[1]

There has been significant progress in the development and clinical use of BATs in the last decade. BATs may be derived from an autograft, allograft, or xenograft source and may be combined with various carriers such as sheets, sprays, or powders. BATs may be a single-layer material and consist of only an epidermal or dermal component. Or they may be bilayer consisting of both epidermal and dermal components. Depending on a BAT's specific characteristics, it may intend to provide either temporary or permanent coverage, with most BATs providing temporary wound coverage.

Mount Auburn Hospital, Harvard Medical School, Cambridge, MA 02138, USA
* Corresponding author.
E-mail address: ecook@mah.harvard.edu

Clin Podiatr Med Surg 31 (2014) 89–101
http://dx.doi.org/10.1016/j.cpm.2013.09.010
0891-8422/14/$ – see front matter © 2014 Elsevier Inc. All rights reserved.

podiatric.theclinics.com

Table 1
Epidermal BATs

Product	Description	Application	Best Available Evidence	Sample Size	Study Endpoint	% Healed
Epicel	Autologous keratinocytes from skin biopsies on pertrolatum gauze	Full/partial thickness wounds: DFUs, burns, venous ulcers	Carsin et al,[18] retrospective, burns	30	5 y	N/A
Myskin	Cultured autologous keratinocytes imbedded on a silicone sheet w/plasma polymer film	Partial-thickness wounds: DFUs, burns	Moustafa et al,[17] prospective, DFUs	16	18 wk	42
Epidex	Autologous keratinocytes from hair follicles on a silicone membrane	Full/partial thickness wounds: burns, venous, DFUs	Ortega-Zilic et al,[20] prospective, mixed etiology	68	9 mo	78

BATs may have inductive properties, meaning that they contain living cells. Some BATs may have scaffolding or conductive properties depending on their characteristics. But a perfect BAT does not yet exist, and the physician must decide which characteristics are desired for a particular wound.[1]

Fully understanding the different available BAT characteristics can reduce overuse by clinicians. Clinically, all BATs need to comply with several major requirements. They should be safe, nontoxic, and nonimmunogenic and have low to no level of transmissible disease to the patient. They should be easy to handle and apply and be able to conform to an irregular recipient wound bed. Ideally they should supplement the integral local environment with a support conduit and growth factors crucial in the healing process. Other characteristics of an ideal BAT are an ability to withstand shear forces for the plantar foot, high durability with varying thicknesses available, and ability to resist infection. An ideal BAT would also need to be cost effective with a long shelf life and easy storage. To date, there is no ideal BAT that meets every above-mentioned characteristic. The treating physician must therefore decide which characteristics are essential when the decision has been made to use a BAT.

When is the use of a BAT justified? Kim and colleagues[1] assert the importance of timing when using these products, emphasizing the question of "are we using these BATs during the proper stage of wound healing?"[1] To answer this question, it is essential to understand when a wound becomes static enough to warrant adjunctive therapy. Sheehan and colleagues[2] suggested that an inadequately healing wound will have a percentage of area reduction less than 10% to 15% per week or less than 50% over the course of a month. There may also be other times when a BAT is warranted. Surgeons may choose to move up or down the reconstructive soft tissue ladder when patient comorbidities or other unique situations make autografts or other standard therapies less desirable.

The fundamental principles in the treatment of chronic diabetic wounds such as debridement and offloading, as discussed in the previous articles, must also be followed when using BATs. The wound environment is crucial to the success of these BATs. Inadequate blood flow, presence of infection, and increased concentration of collagenases or proteases can inhibit the success of any BAT.[3] DFUs are prone to infections and resistant biofilms secondary to a decrease in activity of leukocyte function and migration.[4] An opportunistic local bacterial infection will have further deleterious effects on wound healing, resulting in increased morbidity and mortality.[3] In addition, neuropathy plays a role in reducing the levels of neuropeptides leading to a reduction of capillary blood flow.[5]

Other local mechanisms are also compromised in the chronic diabetic foot ulcer. Research has found that fibroblasts in a chronic nonhealing DFU differ from fibroblasts from those found in an age-matched diabetic control without ulceration. The compromised host has fibroblasts that are less responsive to growth factor signaling and have a deficiency in proliferation. Similarly, keratinocytes, another important cellular component of healing, suffer from impairment of migration and activation in the setting of diabetic wounds. BATs represent a class of adjunctive wound care intended to supplement or replace the extracellular matrix and provide additional growth factors and live or absent fibroblasts, invite cytokines, and provide additional keratinocytes that can promote angiogenesis and cellular proliferation.[5]

A major systemic factor intrinsic to the diabetic state itself is the role of hyperglycemia. Inadequate glycemic control has been indicted by negatively influencing overall healing via increased formation of advanced glycosylation end products. The mechanism is thought to occur by up-regulating the activity of matrix metalloproteinases, which, in turn, inhibits extracellular matrix deposition.[3,6] Over a protracted period, this hyperglycemic state shifts the balance between reactive oxygen species and diminishes the protective antioxidant capacity of the periwound tissue, thus increasing free radical destruction of peripheral cells.[3] The wound becomes mired in the inflammatory phase of healing and results in a buildup of proteolytic enzymes that inhibit or damage local cells attempting to form a new matrix. Cellular apoptosis contributes to and exacerbates the existing wound bioburden promoting an environment susceptible to overt bacterial colonization. A more in-depth review of these factors is beyond the scope of this article.

CLASSIFICATIONS OF BATS

Not all BATs are equal. Understanding how BATs mimic various skin functions is crucial before clinical application. Because of the common misuse of these products, we found a need to simplify and create a classification scheme to aid the clinician in selecting the appropriate BATs for the treatment of DFU. Several classifications systems are used in the literature to stratify bioengineered alternative tissues. These BATs have been classified based on duration of coverage, type of biomaterial, tissue composition regarding cellular component, primary biomaterial preparation (ie, in vitro or in vivo), and the anatomic structure they mimic.[7] In a previous issue of this publication, these BATs were divided among living tissues and bioactive adjuncts.[1] For simplicity, we stratified BATs according to structural composition: epidermal, dermal, and bilayer (dermal/epidermal) with the subcategory of cellular and acellular for each type (**Fig. 1**). This classification of BATs is by no means all inclusive. It is intended to provide a basic framework for understanding a complex process. Although the focus of this article is BATs in the treatment of DFUs, much of the evidence base discusses their use for wounds of various etiologies such as venous, pressure, burns, and ischemic ulcers.

Information is presented in terms of best available evidence. In some instances, a study of a BAT in DFUs may not be available, and their performance in nondiabetic

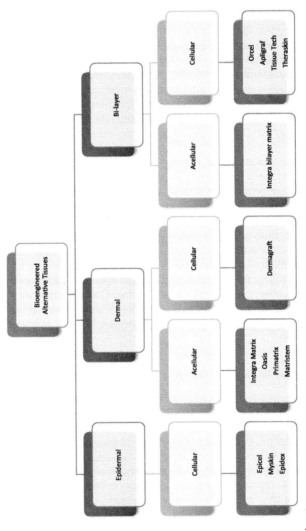

Fig. 1. BAT classification tree.

ulceration populations is presented instead. Brand names are used for literary efficiency and provider recognition. No product or products are explicitly endorsed by the authors.

Each product interacts with the wound environment differently. The evidence base for this topic is extensive, and, as a result, there are many ways that investigators characterize successful and failed outcomes. For the purposes of this article, we discuss the outcomes of BATs in a variety of terms. The simplest and perhaps most clinically relevant is wound healing. The investigators defined the proportion of ulcers that achieved complete healing by a reported time point. Another commonly discussed outcome is designated as tissue "take." In this way, investigators liken the BATs to skin and tissue grafts, which reflect their incorporation into the wound bed. This latter concept is an interesting consideration. First, it supports the role of BATs as a graft substitute. Second, by stratifying the degree of incorporation, investigators bring into question the idea of adequate therapy. For example, if a BAT has a take of 50%, then does that suggest that only 50% of the recipient wound bed received the complete adjunctive treatment? This is question that we leave to you, the reader, to decide for yourself.

The risks that are associated with BATs are more related to whether they are cellular or acellular. Host-graft rejection is a rare occurrence with BATs because cultured epidermal cells do not express major histocompatibility class II human leukocyte antigen–D-related antigens.[7] Many of the dermal scaffold substitutes are acellular; however, there are advantages and disadvantages for each type. Some of these advantages for these acellular products include factors like limited immune response. Acellular products provide the scaffold needed to become vascularized; they also engage with the patient's own fibroblasts and endothelial cells to enhance cellular migration and proliferation.[8] Acellular products are more favorable in that an end user can use it right off the shelf. Despite the ease of access and the lack immunogenic response, there are limitations to using acellular BATs. Tremblay and colleagues[9] found that in mouse models, the overall rate of vascularization was more pronounced with cellular dermal products than acellular substitutes. Cellular BATs benefit from early releases of various growth factors and cytokines that support cellular proliferation.[10] Yannas[11] provided evidence that the presence of living dermal fibroblasts in cellular dermal substitutes lead to better overall wound healing potential with less myofibroblastic activity.

To date, no clinical trial have made head-to-head comparisons of the efficacy of bioengineered extracellular matrix containing live cellular elements verses a product with acellular extracellular matrix. In a proposed study by Lev-Tov and colleagues[12] the investigators will compare Dermagraft (Advanced Tissue Sciences La Jolla, California) with Oasis (Healthpoint Biotherapeutics Texas, USA), with the primary outcome being the percentage of subjects achieving complete would closure by the standard 12 weeks. This study's stated objective is to provide further insight into the cost-to-benefit ratio for the use of cellular verses acellular dermal products in the treatment of chronic diabetic foot ulcers.

Epidermal BATs

Epidermal BATs are derived from a patient's or donor's skin that then undergoes in vitro culturing of the biopsied keratinocytes. Once the keratinocytes are cultured enough, they can be combined into multiple layered sheets. They are known as *cultured epithelial autografts* (CEA) when taken from a patient's own skin. Most epidermal BATs are CEAs because keratinocytes tend to be more immunogenic. Epidermal BATs intend to provide a permanent wound closure but require a dermal matrix if full-thickness wound healing is required.[6] Otherwise, they are fragile and cannot withstand any significant force. These products were originally used to treat burn victims and functioned to form a protective barrier and help prevent sepsis.

CEAs are subdivided into holoclones, meroclones, and paraclones, with holoclones and meroclones having the greatest growth potential before senescence and paraclones with only 15 divisions before cell arrest.[13] The whole culturing process takes approximately 3 to 4 weeks but depends on the amount of cells needed.[14] The most common ways epidermal grafts are delivered include (1) a confluent sheet of cells in which the keratinocytes are allowed, with ample time, to fully differentiate into sheets and then are transferred directly onto the wound bed and (2) growing cells directly on a transfer vehicle; this process allows cells to fully differentiate in vivo. Various delivery vehicles are available for these subconfluent cells, including synthetic membranes, sheets, bovine collagen, aerosol sprays, and microcarrier beads. The advantages of this delivery method include decrease culture time, ease of handling, and application and avoidance of exposure to enzymes involved in the CEA process.[15] The major limitations associated with epidermal BATs are their costs, extended culture time, fragility, and variable incorporation rates ranging from 15% to 85%.[16]

Myskin (Altrika, SO, United Kingdom) is a specific BAT that consists of keratinocytes grown in a silicone vehicle. The current indications for Myskin include diabetic, neuropathic, and pressure ulcerations. The strongest evidence in support of its use is a prospective, randomized, single-blinded control study conducted by Moustafa and colleagues[17] in 2007. This study found a 42% healing rate in an 18-week period with a sample size of 16. Another epidermal substitute, Epicel (Genzyme Biosurgery, Massachusetts, USA), is manufactured using the patient's own keratinocytes harvested from a biopsy. These keratinocytes are cultured to form sheets of CEAs and then directly placed on the wound bed as one confluent sheet. A retrospective study in 2000 by Carsin and colleagues[18] showed good outcomes for burn victims. Another CEA, Epidex (Täfernstrasse, Baden-Dättwil), is obtained from the outer root sheath of the donor's hair follicles that are then grown to form confluent CEA sheets embedded on a silicone membrane.[19] This product is indicated for partial and full-thickness burns and venous and diabetic ulcers. The largest study was conducted in 2010 by Orteg-Zilic and colleagues[20] in a prospective, randomized fashion and showed a 78% healing rate in ulcers of mixed etiology over a 9-month period.

Dermal BATs

The most widely utilized BATs in diabetic foot ulcers are dermal BATs. Because dermal components such as fibroblasts are generally less immunogenic than keratinocytes, most dermal BATs are acellular allografts or xenografts. This allows for reproducible batches that are easier and cheaper to manufacture. Acellular dermal BATs are therefore less expensive and can be made in large reproducible quantities with longer shelf lives. However, randomized controlled trials and well-designed comparative effectiveness studies are severely lacking.

Dermagraft (Advanced Tissue Sciences, California, USA) is one of the few dermal BATs with living cells. More specifically, Dermagraft is an allograft containing living cryopreserved human fibroblasts. Human neonatal (allogeneic) dermal fibroblasts are cultured in vitro onto a biodegradable scaffold.[21] After implantation, the 3-dimensional scaffold allows the fibroblasts to preform signaling pathways, secrete matrix proteins, and release growth factors into the wound milieu that facilitates epithelial migration.

The first phase 3 Dermagraft trial enrolled 281 subjects and did not find a significant reduction in proportion of healed wounds in 12 weeks. However, the second pivotal trial conducted by Marston and colleagues[22] enrolled 314 subjects in a randomized, prospective, multicenter trial in which bioengineered dermal substitute (Dermagraft) was compared with conventional therapy. The inclusion criteria included patients who were diabetic and had a chronic nonhealing plantar ulcer that was present for greater than 6 weeks. These patients had palpable pulses with evidence of necrotic free healthy vascularized wound bed. The study indicated that Dermagraft resulted in complete wound closure in a significantly shorter time along with a significantly lower safety profile compared with the control group. The results indicated an increase in the number of healed wounds at 12 weeks, 30% of which had reported closure using Dermagraft compared with the 18.3% reported closure with standard saline-moistened gauze therapy.

There are many acellular dermal BATs (**Tables 2** and **3**) given their relative ease in production. Oasis is derived from decellularized porcine jejunal submucosa that has been extensively studied in preclinical models. It has been used clinically with diabetic ulcer indications, but the RCT studies are mainly for venous leg ulcers. In a randomized controlled trial, Mostow and colleagues[23] compared the effectiveness of Oasis with that of standard compression therapy alone in the proportion of healed ulcers at 12 weeks. After 12 weeks of treatment, 55% of the wounds treated with Oasis and 34% of the wounds treated with the standard compression therapy healed.[23]

PriMatrix (TEI Biosciences, Massachusetts, USA) is a bioactive acellular dermal tissue matrix derived from fetal bovine skin composed of type I and III collagen. It carries a long shelf life and can be stored at room temperature. Karr[24] in 2011 retrospectively compared wound healing outcomes in 48 diabetic foot or venous stasis wounds who received either PriMatrix or Apligraf (Organogenesis Inc, Massachusetts, USA). Although comparative studies are needed, the method of comparison between the 2 treatment arms was inherently flawed, and drawing valid conclusions is difficult.

Another acellular dermal BAT used in DFUs is GraftJacket (KCI, Texas, USA). GraftJacket is derived from cadaveric skin that undergoes a proprietary process to remove epidermal and dermal cells leaving a dermal matrix. It has a higher type I collagen content than some of its competitors, which increases strength, but the impact of wound incorporation has not been well studied. The best available evidence for GraftJacket was a randomized controlled trial of 86 full-thickness diabetic foot wounds. The absolute difference in time to wound healing between GraftJacket and standard therapy was 1.1 weeks, favoring GraftJacket.[25]

Integra (Integra LifeSciences Corporation New Jersey) is an acellular dermal scaffold that consists of a layer of bovine type 1 collagen chemically altered to include shark glycosaminoglycans (GAG)s and chondroitin 6-sulfate. It is generally classified as a dermal BAT but can also be classified as a bilayered BAT because of the silicone pseudoepithelial layer acting as a protective barrier. At the time of vascularization and neodermis formation, the silicone layer is peeled off within 15 to 20 days.[6] To achieve complete wound closure, the need for an epidermal layer like an Split Thickness Skin Graft (STSG) or a bioengineered alternative is necessary. No randomized controlled trials have been published to date on diabetic foot ulcers. All randomized controlled trials are designed for burn victims with indications for diabetic ulcers. A published retrospective case series by Silverstein reported 5 cases of complete healing with the combination of Integra followed by an STSG.[26]

Bilayer BATs

The last type of BATs on the market is of the bilayer class. Bilayer simply refers to a bioengineered epidermis and dermis together with or without living cells. Several types of bilayer BATs are on the market today. The bilayer breed is more technologically advanced and similar to that of natural skin than any other class of BATs.

Table 2
Dermal BATs

Product	Description	Application	Best Available Evidence	Sample Size	Study Endpoint	% Healed
Dermagraft	Cryopreserved allogeneic neonatal foreskin imbedded in a fibroblast-derived dermal matrix	Full-thickness DFU	Marston et al,[22] prospective, DFUs	314	12 wk	30
Integra matrix	Acellular dermal scaffold w/bovine collagen and chondroitin 6-sulphate (shark derived)	Partial & full-thickness DFU, venous & pressure	Silverstein,[26] retrospective, DFUs	5	Complete healing	100
Oasis	Acellular porcine intestinal submucosa	DFU, venous & pressure	Mostow et al,[23] venous ulcers	120	12 wk	55
Matristem	Acellular porcine bladder-derived single or multilayer extracellular matrix (ECM) sheet	Partial & full-thickness DFU, venous & pressure	Lecheminant & Field, 2012[41], retrospective	34	Complete healing	100
Primatrix	Acellular collagen dermal tissue matrix derived from fetal bovine skin	Full-thickness DFU, venous & pressure	Karr,[24] retrospective, diabetic and venous ulcers	48	Complete healing	100
GraftJacket	Acellular	Full-thickness DFU	Reyzelman et al,[25] randomized controlled trial	86	Time to healing	1.1 wk shorter than standard therapy

Abbreviation: ECM, extracellular matrix.

Table 3
Bilayer (epidermal/dermal) BATs

Product	Description	Application	Best Available Evidence	Sample Size	Study Endpoint	% Healed
Apligraf	Cellular, bovine matrix embedded w/living keratinocytes and fibroblasts NHFFs	DFUs, venous	Veves et al,[31] prospective, DFUs	208	12 wk	56
Integra bilayer	Silicone epidermal substitute over dermal scaffold made of bovine collagen and chondroitin-6-sulphate	Partial and full-thickness DFU, pressure, venous ulcers	Prystowsky et al,[27] retrospective, mixed etiology	16	Complete healing	81
Orcel	Absorbable bovine collagen w/ NHFF-derived fibroblasts & keratinocytes	Venous & DFUs	Trent et al,[28] prospective, venous ulcers	120	12 wk	59
Tissuetech	Combination of Hyalograft 3D and Laserskin	DFUs	Caravaggi et al,[34] prospective, DFUs	79	11 wk	65
Theraskin	Cadaveric allograft derived from STSG w/donor fibroblasts & keratinocytes	DFUs and venous ulcers	Landsman et al,[36] retrospective, DFUs, venous ulcers	188	20 wk	74.5

Abbreviation: NHFF(s), Neonatal Human Foreskin Fibroblast(s).

Because of their complex nature and degree of similar resemblance to normal skin, they are the most expensive when compared with the other BATs.[15]

One of the first and only acellular bilayer products to hit the market in 1981 was Integra. The upper epidermal layer contains a silicone membrane that serves to protect against dehydration and provide flexible coverage of any wound dimension. The second dermal layer contains bovine collagen type I derived from shark chrondroitin-6-sulphate.[15] The objective of this synthetic bilayer BAT is to recruit native host cells to the matrix scaffold, which eventually degrades, and are replaced with newly synthesized host tissue of primarily collagen tissue. Once the wound bed is fully matured, a split-thickness skin graft or epidermal BAT can be used for final closure. In a retrospective study conducted by Prystowsky and colleagues[27] in 2000 using ulcers of mixed etiology, 81% of ulcers healed with a complete to healing endpoint. Orcel (Ortec International Inc New York) is similar in structure to Integra but contains living fibroblasts and keratinocytes imbedded into a lyophilized collagen matrix. It is approved by the US Food and Drug Administration (FDA) for use in burns and blistering skin conditions and not indicated for use in DFUs.[28]

Apligraf, previously known as *Graft Skin*, is another BAT composed of living kerati-nocytes and fibroblasts derived from neonatal foreskin cells.[12] Apligraf is the only cellular bilayer BAT that has FDA approval in the United States for treatment in chronic diabetic foot ulcerations.[29] Unlike human skin, it does not contain blood vessels, hair follicles, sebaceous glands, sweat glands, and cells such as macrophages, melano-cytes, Langerhans's cells, and lymphocytes. Apligraf also has the ability to produce all the cytokines and growth factors found during the normal healing process.[6] Tech-nically, Apligraf is considered a temporary bioactive dressing, as the keratinocytes only last for 1 to 2 months because they are eventually rejected by the host.[30] The strongest study supporting its use was a prospective, randomized, multicenter clinical trial conducted by Veves and colleagues[31] in 2001. It was hypothesized that a weekly application of Apligraf for a maximum of 5 applications would increase the wound healing rate in noninfected, nonischemic, chronic plantar DFUs when compared with saline-moistened gauze. There were 208 diabetic patients with neuropathic wounds. During a 12-week period, a greater number of patients in the Apligraf group (56%) achieved complete wound healing when compared with 38% in the control group. The median time for complete closure was significantly lower for the Apligraf group when compared with the control group at 65 and 90 days, respectively. Since the Veves study, there have been several other investigations limited to case series or studies with retrospective small sample sizes, which reported similar outcomes.[32] A major limitation to Apligraf is its shelf life, which is about 5 days, and expense.[6]

Other cellular bilayered BATs include PermaDerm (Regenicin, Inc, New Jersey) and Tissuetech (Bio-Tissue, Inc, Florida, USA). These BATs contain keratinocytes and fi-broblasts, which give the additional benefit of inducing angiogenic and inflammatory mediators to the site of the ulceration. These BATs contain an upper layer of neonatal human foreskin keratinocytes and a lower layer of bovine-derived collagen matrix implanted with neonatal human foreskin fibroblasts.[15] An observational study by Uccioli[33] in 2003 found a healing rate of 91% in 12 weeks with the use of Tissuetech in the treatment of DFUs. A randomized control trial by Caravaggi and colleagues[34] in 2003 also showed a 65% healing rate at 12 weeks. Another retrospective study conducted by Uccioli[35] that included 975 patients with 1156 wounds concluded that Tissuetech was an effective and safe substitute that could provide an improved cost-benefit ratio over time. Another cellular bilayered BAT worth mentioning is Ther-askin, (Soluble Systems, LLC Virginia, USA) a human cadaveric allograft containing donor fibroblasts and keratinocytes. Landsman and colleagues[36] conducted a pro-spective study in 2011 on diabetic and venous ulcers and showed a 74.5% healing rate in a 20-week period. A Cochrane review in 2007 showed promising results that concluded a place for bilayer BATs in conjunction with the use of compressive ther-apy, which showed an increase venous ulcer-healing rate when compared with using compressive therapy alone with local wound care.[37]

Future of BATs

Current products on the market are targeted at supplementing the existing natural mechanisms of wound repair and are not geared for replacing functions of lost tissues. Most nonautologous BATs predominantly function as a bioactive dressing. The BATs composed primarily of autologous keratinocytes and fibroblasts show more promising results in randomized controlled trials.[6] There are many obstacles to developing sub-stitutes that closely mimic all the functions of natural skin. Some of these functions include viscoelastic properties, pigmentation, sweat glands, and tactile sensation. Contemporary BATs can only replace the protective barrier function of skin.[6] Tissue regeneration, as seen in injured reptiles and starfish, have provided clues in nature that tissue can fully regenerate. Similar examples in humans include the regeneration of liver tissue after injury.

Embryonic stem cell research is in its infancy and has been delayed because of ethical and political debates. However, recent investigations consider the use of adult stem cells for skin regeneration.[38] In an in vitro study, bone marrow–derived stem cells are shown to synthesize higher amounts of collagen, growth factors, and angiogenic factors compared with native dermal fibroblasts, which may be associated with accelerated wound healing.[39] The holy grail of tissue replacement has yet to be discovered. Nevertheless, if researchers and bioengineers can flip the switch to return cells to their prenatal period, this, in fact, can be a real breakthrough in cellular regeneration. In 2007, Yamanaka,[40] was the first to reprogram the cell back to its embryonic state by introducing 4 genes (Oct-3/4, Sox2, c-Myc, and KLF4) into a human skin cell. In the postnatal period, the human cannot regenerate skin tissue, only unorganized scar tissue. However, in the early prenatal period, when injury to all skin layers or appendages occurrs, the embryo can fully regenerate identical functional tissue and not scar tissue.[11]

REFERENCES

1. Kim PJ, Heilala M, Steinberg JS, et al. Bioengineered alternative tissues and hyperbaric oxygen in lower extremity wound healing. Clin Podiatr Med Surg 2007; 24(3):529–46 x. Available at: http://www.ncbi.nlm.nih.gov/pubmed/17613390. Accessed July 6, 2013.
2. Sheehan P, Jones P, Caselli A. Percent Change in wound area of diabetic foot ulcers over a 4-week period is a robust predictor of complete healing in a 12-week prospective trial. Diabetes Care 2003;26(6):1879–82.
3. Gary Sibbald R, Woo KY. The biology of chronic foot ulcers in persons with diabetes. Diabetes Metab Res Rev 2008;24(Suppl 1):25–30.
4. Neut D, Tijdens-Creusen EJ, Bulstra SK, et al. Biofilms in chronic diabetic foot ulcers–a study of 2 cases. Acta Orthop 2011;82(3):383–5. Available at: http://www.pubmedcentral.nih.gov/articlerender.fcgi?artid=3235322&tool=pmcentrez&rendertype=abstract. Accessed July 14, 2013.
5. Loots MA, Lamme EN, Zeegelaar J, et al. Differences in cellular infiltrate and extracellular matrix of chronic diabetic and venous ulcers versus acute wounds. J Invest Dermatol 1998;111(5):850–7. Available at: http://www.ncbi.nlm.nih.gov/pubmed/9804349.
6. Shevchenko RV, James SL, James SE. A review of tissue-engineered skin bioconstructs available for skin reconstruction. J R Soc Interface 2010;7(43): 229–58. Available at: http://www.pubmedcentral.nih.gov/articlerender.fcgi?artid=2842616&tool=pmcentrez&rendertype=abstract.
7. Hefton JM, Madden MR, Finkelstein JL, et al. Grafting of burn patients with allografts of cultured epidermal cells. Lancet 1983;2(8347):428–30.
8. Lazic T, Falanga V. Bioengineered skin constructs and their use in wound healing. Plast Reconstr Surg 2011;127(Suppl 1):75S–90S.
9. Tremblay PL, Hudon V, Berthod F, et al. Inosculation of tissue-engineered capillaries with the host's vasculature in a reconstructed skin transplanted on mice. Am J Transplant 2005;5(5):1002–10.
10. Ehrenreich M, Ruszczak Z. Update on tissue-engineered biological dressings. Tissue Eng 2006;12(9):2407–24.
11. Yannas IV. Similarities and differences between induced organ regeneration in adults and early fetal regeneration. J R Soc Interface 2005;2(10):403–17.

12. Lev-Tov H, Li CS, Dahle S, et al. Cellular versus acellular matrix devices in treatment of diabetic foot ulcers: study protocol for a comparative efficacy randomized controlled trial. Trials 2013;14:8. Available at: http://www.pubmedcentral.nih.gov/articlerender.fcgi?artid=3553036&tool=pmcentrez&rendertype=abstract.

13. Atiyeh BS, Costagliola M. Cultured epithelial autograft (CEA) in burn treatment: three decades later. Burns 2007;33(4):405–13. Available at: http://www.ncbi.nlm.nih.gov/pubmed/17400392. Accessed May 23, 2013.

14. Chester DL, Balderson DS, Papini RP. A review of keratinocyte delivery to the wound bed. J Burn Care Rehabil 2004;25:266–75, 12.

15. Greaves NS, Iqbal SA, Baguneid M, et al. The role of skin substitutes in the management of chronic cutaneous wounds. Wound Repair Regen 2013;21(2):194–210. Available at: http://www.ncbi.nlm.nih.gov/pubmed/23437811. Accessed June 4, 2013.

16. Williamson JS, Snelling CF, Clugston P, et al. Cultured epithelial autograft: five years of clinical experience with 28 patients. J Trauma 1995;39(2):309–19.

17. Moustafa M, Bullock A, Creagh F, et al. A Randomised controlled single blind prospective pilot study on the use of autologous keratinocytes on a transfer dressing (Myskin) in the treatment of non-healing diabetic ulcers. Regen Med 2007;2:887–902.

18. Carsin H, Ainaud P, Le Bever H, et al. Cultured epithelial autografts in extensive burn coverage of severely traumatized patients: a five year single-center experience with 30 patients. Burns 2000;26(4):379–87.

19. Tausche AK. An autologous epidermal equivalent tissue-engineered from follicular outer root sheath keratinocytes is as effective as split-thickness skin autograft in recalcitrant vascular leg ulcers. Wound Repair Regen 2003;11:248–52.

20. Ortega-Zilic N, Hunziker T, Lauchli S, et al. Epidex Swiss field trial 2004-2008. Dermatology 2010;221:365–72.

21. Marston WA. Dermagraft, a bioengineered human dermal equivalent for the treatment of chronic nonhealing diabetic foot ulcer. Expert Rev Med Devices 2004;1(1):21–31. Available at: http://www.ncbi.nlm.nih.gov/pubmed/16293007.

22. Marston W, Hanft J, Norwood P, et al. The efficacy and safety of Dermagraft in improving the healing of chronic diabetic foot ulcers: results of a prospective randomized trial. Diabetes Care 2003;26(6):1701–5.

23. Mostow EN, Haraway GD, Dalsing M, et al. Effectiveness of an extracellular matrix graft (OASIS Wound Matrix) in the treatment of chronic leg ulcers: a randomized clinical trial. J Vasc Surg 2005;41(5):837–43. Available at: http://www.ncbi.nlm.nih.gov/pubmed/15886669. Accessed July 13, 2013.

24. Karr J. Retrospective comparison of diabetic foot ulcer and venous stasis ulcer healing outcome between a dermal repair scaffold (Primatrix) and a bilayered living cell therapy (Apligraf). Adv Skin Wound Care 2011;24:119–25.

25. Reyzelman A, Crews RT, Moore JC, et al. Clinical effectiveness of an acellular dermal regenerative tissue matrix compared to standard wound management in healing diabetic foot ulcers: a prospective, randomized, multicenter study. Int Wound J 2009;6(3):196–208, 20.

26. Silverstein G. Dermal regeneration template in the surgical management of diabetic foot ulcers: a series of five cases. J Foot Ankle Surg 2006;45(1):28–33. Available at: http://www.ncbi.nlm.nih.gov/pubmed/16399556. Accessed July 6, 2013.

27. Prystowsky J, Nowygrod R, Marboe C, et al. Artificial Skin (Integra Dermal Regeneration Template) for closure of lower extremity wounds. Vasc Endovasc Surg 2000;34:557–67.

28. Trent J, Falabella A, Eaglstein WH, et al. Venous ulcers: pathophysiology and treatment options. Ostomy Wound Manage 2005;51:38–54.

29. Widgerow AD. Bioengineered skin substitute considerations in the diabetic foot ulcer. Ann Plast Surg 2013 [Epub ahead of print]. Available at: http://www.ncbi.nlm.nih.gov/pubmed/23511743. Accessed June 7, 2013.

30. Clark RA, Ghosh K, Tonnesen MG. Tissue engineering for cutaneous wounds. J Invest Dermatol 2007;127(5):1018–29.

31. Veves A, Falanga V, Armstrong DG, et al. Graftskin, a human skin equivalent. Diabetes Care 2001;24(2):290–5.

32. Curran MP, Plosker GL. Bilayered bioengineered skin a review of its use in the treatment of venous leg ulcers and diabetic foot ulcers. BioDrugs 2002;16(6):439–55.

33. Uccioli L. Clinical results realted to the use of TissueTech autograft system in the treatment of diabetic foot ulceration. Wounds 2003;15:279–88.

34. Caravaggi C, Giglio R, Pritelli C, et al. HYAFF 11 – based autologous dermal and epidermal grafts in the treatment of noninfected diabetic plantar and dorsal. Diabetes Care 2003;26(10):2853–9.

35. Uccioli L. A clinical investigation on the characteristics and outcomes of treating chronic lower extremity wounds using the tissuetech autograft system. Int J Low Extrem Wounds 2003;2:140–51.

36. Landsman A, Cook J, Cook E, et al. A retrospective clinical study of 188 consecutive patients to examine the effectiveness of a biological active cryopreserved human skin allograft(Theraskin) on the treatment of diabetic ulcers and venous leg ulcers. Foot Ankle Spec 2011;4:29–41.

37. Jones J, Nelson E. Skin grafting for venous leg ulcers. Cochrane Database Syst Rev 2007;(2):CD00173.

38. Nakagawa H, Akita S, Fukui M, et al. Human mesenchymal stem cells successfully improve skin-substitute wound healing. Br J Dermatol 2005;153(1):29–36.

39. Han SK, Yoon TH, Lee DG, et al. Potential of human bone marrow stromal cells to accelerate wound healing in vitro. Ann Plast Surg 2005;55(4):414–9.

40. Yamanaka S. Strategies and new developments in the generation of patient-specific pluripotent stem cells. Cell Stem Cell 2007;1(1):39–49.

41. Lecheminant J, Field C. Porcine Urinary Bladder Matrix: A Retrospective Study and Establishment of Protocol. Journal of Wound Care 2012;21(10):476–82.

Partial Foot Amputations for Salvage of the Diabetic Lower Extremity

Troy J. Boffeli, DPM, FACFAS*, Jonathan C. Thompson, DPM, MHA

KEYWORDS

- Diabetic lower extremity • Partial foot amputation • Lower limb amputation
- Diabetes mellitus

KEY POINTS

- A variety of partial foot amputation procedures exist for salvage of the diabetic lower extremity.
- Procedure selection is based on the extent of nonviable or infected tissue, healing potential from a vascular standpoint, biomechanical functionality, and patient goals.
- The surgical approach for partial foot amputations varies from elective procedures, often requiring staged surgery and a unique surgical technique.
- A subset of patients may be better served with proximal amputation depending on medical comorbidities, ambulatory status, and ultimate patient goals.

INTRODUCTION

Diabetes-related lower extremity ulcers are a common yet unfortunate complication of diabetes mellitus. Fifteen to 25% of diabetic patients are at risk of developing an ulcer during their lifetime, with 15% of these requiring subsequent amputation for infection management.[1–4] Of the approximately 80,000 amputations performed in the United States annually, half of these consist of a below-knee or more proximal amputation.[5] Patients with a below-knee amputation have a 1-year mortality rate between 20.8% and 35.5%,[6,7] with a reported contralateral limb loss rate of 53.3% within 5 years.[8] Furthermore, ambulatory status is decreased in patients with proximal amputations due to inefficient biomechanics leading to increased energy and oxygen demand.[9,10] Thus, partial foot amputation should be attempted when possible to help minimize morbidity and optimize functionality in this high-risk patient population. The principal goals of surgical treatment of diabetes-related foot infection, complicated ulceration, osteomyelitis, or gangrene consist of selecting the appropriate procedure to

Foot and Ankle Surgical Residency Program, Regions Hospital/HealthPartners Institute for Education and Research, 640 Jackson Street, Saint Paul, Minnesota 55101, USA
* Corresponding author.
E-mail address: troy.j.boffeli@healthpartners.com

Clin Podiatr Med Surg 31 (2014) 103–126
http://dx.doi.org/10.1016/j.cpm.2013.09.005
0891-8422/14/$ – see front matter © 2014 Elsevier Inc. All rights reserved.

effectively eradicate nonsalvageable tissue, relieve pain, achieve primary healing, and preserve as much limb length as possible from a functionality standpoint.[11,12] Procedure selection in determining the most appropriate amputation level is typically based on ulcer location, extent of osteomyelitis or gangrene, and biomechanical implications. Local amputation options mainly consist of partial or complete toe, partial or complete ray, transmetatarsal, Lisfranc, Chopart, or Syme amputations. This article discusses each of these amputation procedures in a distal to proximal fashion, with ray amputations being stratified into first and fifth ray, or border ray, amputation and central ray amputation, as the surgical approach varies between these 2 groups. Discussion focuses on procedure selection as well as both standard and advanced surgical techniques in performing partial foot amputations for the prevention of major proximal lower limb amputations.

SURGICAL CONSIDERATIONS

Although surgical management of wounds with underlying soft tissue infection in the diabetic patient must often be addressed in an urgent fashion, careful preoperative planning is of paramount importance. When determining the surgical plan in this setting, consideration must be given to the location and extent of ulceration, infection, or gangrene, healing potential from a vascular standpoint, and the implications of a particular partial foot amputation on biomechanical function. The necessary laboratory, imaging, and, when appropriate, vascular studies should routinely be correlated with clinical findings. A single-stage amputation with immediate closure is possible when osteomyelitis is present without associated abscess or cellulitis, but acute soft tissue infection often requires a staged surgical approach. The surgeon should not feel compelled to solve complex diabetes-related foot infections with a single surgery. Staged surgery can oftentimes lead to better results with fewer complications than nonstaged surgery. The optimal definitive incision plan can be drawn out before making the stage 1 incision to ensure that the initial incision and drainage procedure will not compromise subsequent closure options. The first-stage procedure typically involves excision of the ulcer and surrounding necrotic tissue, incision and drainage of any abscess, resection of bone, and bone biopsy, as needed, to allow resolution of soft tissue infection. Multiple incision and drainage procedures may be necessary every couple of days in the setting of persistent cellulitis, abscess, or unresolving leukocytosis. Final-stage treatment occurs once the soft tissue infection has resolved and involves thorough irrigation and debridement, raising a flap if necessary, resection of previous incision borders, final proximal margin bone biopsy, and tension-free closure.

The incision and dissection technique in wound, flap, and amputation surgery differs from typical elective foot surgery because of the increased concern for maintaining tissue viability, decreased concern for sensory nerves, and salvage nature of diabetic foot surgery. The incision is made full-thickness with the scalpel plunging down to bone at a 90-degree angle to the skin surface in an attempt to avoid skiving or undermining skin edges, which could compromise viability of the local soft tissue and healing potential (**Fig. 1**). The scalpel is then advanced using a vertical sawing motion. The skin should be in a relaxed, tension-free position when performing the incision to avoid creating a serrated wound edge. This is particularly important at certain amputation sites, such as incising between the toes in a digital amputation. Longitudinal tension applied in line with the incision can also be helpful in creating a smooth incision. No undermining or layered dissection is typically performed, as this can act to devitalize tissues. Dissection should be full-thickness in nature whenever possible, with tissue

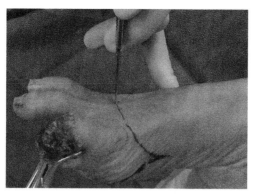

Fig. 1. Amputation surgery incisional technique contrasts from other surgical procedures, requiring a full-thickness incision made at 90° to the skin surface. This minimizes the tendency to bevel the incision or prematurely undermine the flap.

flaps raised at a level below the periosteum. Excessive periosteal stripping beyond the level of bone resection should be avoided, as this can be detrimental to osseous blood supply and possibly increase the likelihood of heterotopic ossification (HO) formation. HO formation is a relatively common but overlooked complication of wound surgery that can lead to reulceration when it forms on the weight-bearing surface in the neuropathic foot. We have appreciated a higher tendency toward HO formation in younger patients with diabetic ulcer who typically have a combination of profound neuropathy and robust blood supply. The most common site where we have seen clinically relevant HO formation with associated reulceration is with amputations involving partial metatarsal resection (**Fig. 2**). We routinely refer high-risk patients, particularly those with past history of heterotopic bone formation, to a radiation therapy specialist for 1-time prophylactic radiation treatment within 24 hours preoperatively to 72 hours postoperatively. This is an effective treatment adjunct with a recurrence rate of 18% in patients with previous heterotopic bone growth at our institution.[13]

Most diabetes-related neuropathic foot ulcers are related to underlying structural deformity or biomechanical issues, which need to be identified and addressed if partial foot amputation is to be successful. For instance, partial foot amputation for a forefoot ulcer caused by ankle equinus will likely fail if the equinus is not surgically addressed either at the time of amputation or as a delayed procedure if infection raises concern for cross-contamination.

Neuropathic ulcerations with underlying osteomyelitis secondary to structural deformity are often treated with excision of the infected bone. This may be done through the excised ulcer or through a separate incision while the ulceration is allowed to heal secondarily. In contrast, local amputation flap techniques allow complete closure of the wound with viable tissue. Advanced amputation techniques using local rotational and advancement flaps may also allow for more distal resection than standard amputation techniques, thus better preserving biomechanical function and cosmesis. Flap construction often requires increased planning, applying basic plastic surgery principles. Knowledge of foot and ankle angiosome principles is important because amputation-related flaps generally involve the medial or lateral plantar artery angiosomes. The ideal amputation flap technique uses soft tissue that would otherwise be discarded with traditional amputation techniques. In doing so, flap construction will not compromise revision options in the event of flap failure. Flaps are to be created in full-thickness fashion without undermining or layered dissection. A

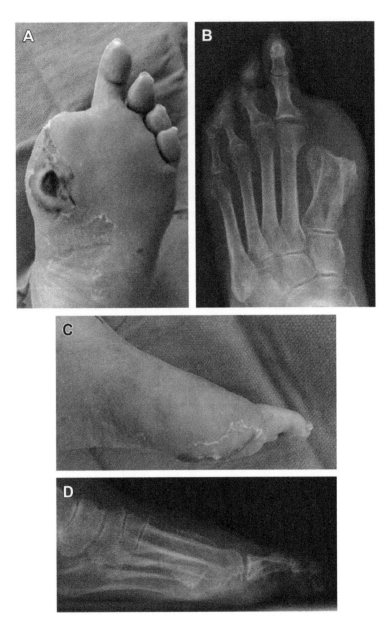

Fig. 2. (A–D) Heterotopic ossification formation can complicate partial foot amputations and has the potential to cause recurrent neuropathic ulceration.

minimal-touch technique should be used while handling the flap. Surgery involving flap closure is oftentimes performed in a staged manner, and closure is not performed until resolution of acute infection is appreciated. Delayed flap closure after initial debridement minimizes the likelihood of complicating hematoma formation and provides seemingly better resolution of the infectious process. Flap planning in staged surgery should start before the initial open amputation or incision and drainage procedure in an effort to preserve viable tissue for subsequent closure.

Maintaining effective hemostasis is of central importance to minimize the potential for excessive blood loss or hematoma formation. Procedures are often performed without a tourniquet to help determine viable versus nonviable tissue and better visualize bleeding vessels for ligation. A tourniquet can be applied but not inflated initially if concern exists for excessive bleeding compromising the surgical field. Although small vessels can be electrocauterized, moderate to large vessels should be ligated with absorbable hand-ties to maintain hemostasis yet avoid excessive tissue devitalization. Electrocautery is mainly used for selective local hemostasis, as opposed to widespread hemostasis or dissection. Minimal diffuse bleeding can often be contained by a tamponade effect with closure, but if concern exists for hematoma formation, a closed-suction drain should be placed or, alternately, the wound packed open and treated with a topical thrombotic agent. Drain removal can be performed once output has significantly reduced, typically on the first or second day postoperatively.

Closure technique in wound and amputation surgery is often critical to the success of the procedure. Deep closure with absorbable suture can be variably performed depending on the amputation level, as this may help decrease dead space and remove tension from the skin closure site. Excessive deep or layered closure should be avoided, especially when tissue viability is marginal or the potential for persistent infection exists. Routine skin closure is performed in full-thickness fashion with interrupted sutures, with care being taken to avoid excessive tension on the local soft tissues. This may require using temporary or interval retention sutures during closure. A nonabsorbable, unbraided suture is typically recommended to avoid harboring detrimental bacteria. Sutures may be left intact for an extended period as compared with elective foot surgery, often remaining in place for up to 4 to 6 weeks depending on the location of the surgical wound, healing progress, and quality of surrounding tissues.

FIRST RAY AMPUTATION
Hallux Distal Syme Amputation

Tip-of-toe distal hallux amputation may be performed in the setting of distal ulcerations complicated by osteomyelitis in the distal phalanx. Ulceration of the distal tip of the hallux is often seen in the setting of hallux malleus or hammertoe deformity, whereas a dystrophic toenail could lead to resultant ulceration as well. Maintaining maximal length to the hallux is desirable from a patient satisfaction standpoint, as well as for optimal preservation of first ray function. When osteomyelitis is contained to the distal phalanx, a hallux distal Syme amputation is a viable option to eradicate infection, excise the ulcer, correct digital deformity, and permanently remove the toenail while maintaining length for improved cosmesis and dynamic function. A transverse fishmouth incision is performed with medial and lateral apices slightly proximal to the interphalangeal joint (IPJ). The proximal extent of the toenail matrix limits available length of the dorsal flap, and care is taken to incise sufficiently proximal to avoid regrowth of nail material. The plantar flap is limited only by the size and location of the ulcer and is typically longer than the dorsal flap, which creates a mismatched incision length and frequently causes a slight pucker between sutures. This can be mitigated by lowering the medial and lateral apices to increase the dorsal flap size. Disarticulation is performed at the IPJ, and the specimen is transferred to the back table for later processing. This helps isolate infection from the proximal margin specimen that will subsequently be obtained. The head of the proximal phalanx is then remodeled to remove prominences by resecting the metaphyseal flares and plantar condyles (**Fig. 3**). Care is taken to preserve as much bone length as possible without increasing risk of reulceration. Distal phalanx resection provides bone for biopsy while the

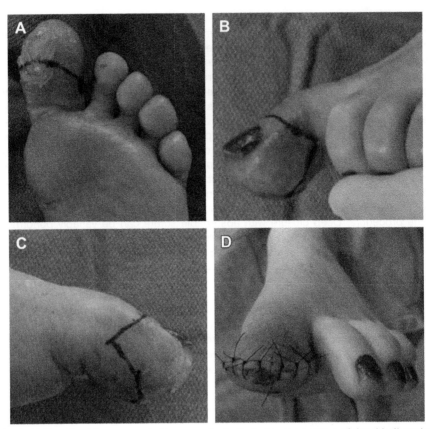

Fig. 3. Hallux distal Syme amputations may be indicated in the setting of distal hallux ulcer complicated by osteomyelitis. (*A–C*) Incision planning for hallux distal Syme amputation. (*D*) Minimal tension is appreciated with closure.

remodeled proximal phalanx allows margin biopsy that is typically clear of osteomyelitis from a pathologic standpoint. Closure is performed with full-thickness interrupted sutures. The patient is allowed to weight bear in a postoperative shoe until sutures are removed, typically at 3 to 4 weeks postoperatively.

Hallux Amputation

Although hallux distal Syme amputation is indicated for tip of toe ulcers, partial or complete hallux amputation is typically used for plantar IPJ ulcers. The location of ulcerated tissue, extent of infected bone, mechanical abnormalities, and viability of local soft tissue largely determine the level of amputation with first ray and other foot amputation procedures. Plantar hallux IPJ neuropathic ulcerations frequently lead to infection of the proximal phalanx and commonly occur due to an underlying hallux rigidus deformity or prominent plantar IPJ sesamoid that increases plantar hallux pressure. Plantar medial IPJ ulcerations can develop due to an excessive valgus attitude of the hallux secondary to severe flatfoot deformity or hallux valgus. Potential also exists for dorsal IPJ ulceration secondary to a hallux malleus or hammertoe deformity. Once osteomelitis develops, nonhealing IPJ ulcers complicated by these mechanical and structural deformities are often treated with hallux amputation. Reconstructive procedures to correct deformities contributing to ulceration are also effective but should be considered before the development of abscess and osteomyelitis. Hallux amputation can be performed either by retaining the base of the proximal phalanx or, more commonly, disarticulation at the metatarsophalangeal joint (MPJ). Retaining the metatarsal head is possible for ulcers located at the IPJ to maintain a functional sesamoid apparatus and minimize the likelihood of transfer lesions at the second MPJ. When selecting between these procedure options, consideration should be given to any underlying structural deformity of the foot so as to choose an amputation level that will minimize the likelihood of reulceration. A full-thickness transverse fish-mouth incision is commonly used, with dorsal and plantar flaps ideally of similar length extending to the middle of the proximal phalanx (**Fig. 4**A–B). Care should be taken when planning the flaps, as a shorter flap will place excessive tension on the incision with closure, whereas a longer flap will increase dead space at the amputation site, thus increasing the possibility of hematoma formation. The lateral convergence of the dorsal and plantar incisions should be located midline on the toe in the sagittal plane. A sharp towel clamp is placed through the distal hallux to promote a no-touch technique and provide effective manipulation during dissection. The soft tissue flap margins are handled with a minimal-touch technique by using a double-pronged skin hook to raise dorsal and plantar flaps in full-thickness fashion. Subperiosteal dissection is performed to the level of the phalangeal resection or MPJ disarticulation. The osteotomy is largely transverse with subtle dorsal-distal to plantar-proximal angulation to prevent a prominent bone margin on the weight-bearing surface when preserving the base of the proximal phalanx. The long extensor tendon distinctly attaches to the skin along the length of the proximal phalanx causing proximal retraction of the

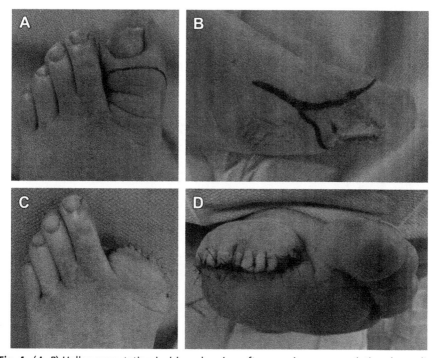

Fig. 4. (*A, B*) Hallux amputation incision planning often requires some variation depending on the location of the ulceration. (*C, D*) Closure of the hallux amputation.

dorsal flap once released from its main attachment on the distal phalanx. Failure to adequately detach and remove the leading edge of this tendon promotes tension on the incision margins and may ultimately be a detriment to healing. The patient is made minimally weight-bearing in a postoperative shoe, and sutures are left in place for 2 to 4 weeks.

Partial or Complete First Ray Resection

Partial first ray resection is typically used to treat diabetic neuropathic ulcers located beneath the first metatarsal head that have become complicated by infection involving cellulitis, abscess, MPJ sepsis, or osteomyelitis. Amputation of the hallux and removal of the first metatarsal head may also be necessary for proximal spread of infection from tip-of-toe and IPJ hallux ulcerations or ulcerated hallux valgus deformities complicated by osteomyelitis. The standard incision for partial first ray amputation involves a tennis racket–type incision, with the proximal arm made midline along the first metatarsal head and neck, creating matching dorsal and plantar flaps. This standard first ray amputation incision works well when the ulcer is located medially on the first metatarsal head within the excised soft tissue, at the hallux IPJ location distal to the plantar incision or when the plantar ulcer is partial thickness and will heal secondarily once the underlying bone is removed. Plantar first MPJ ulcers present a unique challenge in that the standard first ray incision approach does not allow excision and closure of the plantar ulcers without excessive bone resection. Full-thickness neuropathic ulcers on the plantar surface of the foot can be left to heal secondarily after amputation, but this can result in ongoing nonhealing wounds and persistent bone exposure. Isolated metatarsal head resection with ulcer excision and local flap closure can be considered in an effort to preserve the hallux. However, we find the hallux to be destabilized and minimally functional, frequently becoming contracted and at risk for future ulceration. Conversely, partial first ray resection combined with rotational flap closure is a useful option in the setting of plantar metatarsal head ulceration. The first ray flap incision is designed to create a flap from the medial side of the proximal phalanx and first metatarsal head while excising the plantar ulcer (**Fig. 5**). The proximal arm of the incision curves medially away from the weight-bearing surface to extend

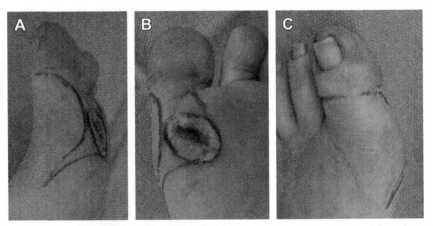

Fig. 5. (A–C) Incision planning for partial first ray amputation with rotational flap closure. Minimal tissue is discarded and much of the digital tissue is preserved to create the rotational flap. This technique allows complete closure of the plantar wound once the first toe and metatarsal head are removed.

along the medial midline of the first metatarsal. This technique minimizes postoperative weight-bearing on the incision and is more easily converted to transmetatarsal amputation (TMA) should that become necessary in the near or distant future. The dorsal flap incision on the hallux is approximately midway along the proximal phalanx and appears transverse when viewed on the dorsal surface of the foot. This transverse hallux incision continues along the lateral side of the toe, preserving the full-thickness digital soft tissue. The flap is raised beneath the periosteum, creating a full-thickness flap of soft tissue, including neurovascular structures, periosteum, extensor tendons, subcutaneous fat, and skin. This is performed with a minimal-touch technique by using a wide double-prong skin hook on the flap and a sharp towel clamp through the distal hallux for ease of manipulation. The hallux is disarticulated at the MPJ, and a bone saw is then used to resect the first metatarsal head just proximal to the distal metaphyseal flare. Care is taken to bevel the metatarsal to avoid prominence at the plantar aspect of the weight-bearing surface or along the medial margin where footwear could rub. The first metatarsal medullary canal is inspected for purulent-appearing medullary bone, which is curetted to healthy bleeding bone. It is not unusual for the entire medullary canal to be abnormal. A significant attempt is made to preserve viable metatarsal cortex just proximal to the distal metaphyseal flare as retaining metatarsal length is beneficial for weight-bearing function. Excessive loss of length may also have negative consequences if later conversion to TMA is necessary. Margin biopsy helps to determine the duration of antibiotics. The flap is then rotated into place and closed without tension.[14]

As an alternative to the traditional open technique common with multiple-stage amputation, the stage 1 procedure may involve preliminary flap closure over antibiotic-impregnated beads. The stage 2 procedure is scheduled 2 weeks later and involves opening of the distal non weight-bearing portion of the flap, antibiotic bead chain removal, hematoma curettage, and clean margin bone biopsy of the first metatarsal. This multiple-stage approach decreases the potential for hematoma and thus HO formation that may otherwise complicate wound healing. It furthermore allows temporary closure before full resolution of cellulitis, effectively shortening hospitalization time and duration of antibiotics. Finally, staged closure with antibiotic-impregnated beads helps preserve flap length and decreases likelihood of contamination of the proximal clean margin bone biopsy. Full-thickness closure is performed with nonabsorbable interrupted sutures. The patient is made non weight-bearing until sutures are removed at 3 to 4 weeks postoperatively, depending on healing progression.

Infrequently, a previous partial first ray amputation stump site can become ulcerated and complicated by osteomyelitis or, alternately, contiguous spread of osteomyelitis from a distal source can extend into the proximal aspect of the first metatarsal, which may necessitate the need for complete first ray amputation. Complete first ray resection should be avoided if possible, as concern exists for tendon imbalance postoperatively secondary to potential disruption of the peroneus longus and tibialis anterior tendon insertion sites. Furthermore, complete first ray resection has the potential to disrupt the midfoot Lisfranc complex and compromise medial column integrity. If subsequent conversion to TMA were necessary, the parabola established by the remaining metatarsals may increase the risk of reulceration beneath the second metatarsal stump site. Preoperative magnetic resonance imaging and intraoperative appearance of the medullary canal help determine the need for partial versus complete first metatarsal amputation. The incision for complete first metatarsal amputation closely resembles the first ray flap technique previously discussed but the proximal arm is extended to the medial midfoot. As the medial incision is extended proximally, care is taken to preserve the attachment of the tibialis anterior tendon into the medial cuneiform. A sharp towel clamp is used to distract the metatarsal in the medial direction while the ligamentous structures and peroneus longus are sharply transected from the lateral base of the first metatarsal. Care is taken to avoid the proximal perforating artery and deep peroneal nerve in the first interspace. The staged antibiotic bead protocol is typically used in this setting, as there is frequently concern for contiguous spread to the midfoot in cases necessitating complete ray amputation. To accommodate the dead space in this region, a helical antibiotic bead chain configuration is used. Similar to the previously discussed protocol, beads are removed in a secondary procedure 2 weeks later. The adjacent medial cuneiform may require minimal contouring with a rongeur at that time to remove prominences, and the resected bone can be processed as a proximal margin biopsy to help direct the duration of antibiotic therapy. The medial cuneiform and second metatarsal base are otherwise left undisturbed. The patient is to remain non weight-bearing for 6 weeks postoperatively to protect the tibialis anterior and peroneus longus tendons. The patient may require indefinite arch support or ankle-foot orthosis use to maximize stability and biomechanical function following surgery.

CENTRAL RAY AMPUTATION
Central Toe Distal Syme Amputation

Central ray amputation techniques often differ from first and fifth border ray amputations. Border rays are defined as the first and fifth ray whereas central rays are considered the second, third, and fourth rays. Diabetes-related tip of central toe ulcers are typically associated with underlying hammertoe contracture and peripheral neuropathy. Such ulcers are often recurrent or chronic in nature, with osteomyelitis progressing slowly. The combination of digital deformity and neuropathy results in nonhealing, deep sores that frequently become complicated by osteomyelitis. This condition can lead to devastating and very costly limb loss if not identified and treated aggressively in the early stages. Uncomplicated cases can be performed in a minor procedure room in clinic whereas more complicated cases involving proximal spread of cellulitis may require inpatient surgical intervention and care. The standard incision for ulcers at the distal tip of a central toe is a transverse fishmouth incision in full-thickness fashion (**Fig. 6**A–B). An attempt is made to match the dorsal and plantar flap arms to avoid incongruent edges and prominent apical soft tissue redundancy with closure. The plantar flap is inherently larger, as the dorsal flap requires excision of the toenail and matrix. The plantar flap should remain full-thickness as it will be advanced anteriorly with closure, relocating the plantar tissue pulp to the weight-bearing surface. Initial disarticulation at the distal IPJ allows removal of the typically infected distal phalanx, tip-of-toe ulcer, toenail, and nail matrix. The distal one-third of the middle phalanx is removed to allow for clean margin biopsy and tension-free closure. Furthermore, adequate bone resection may intentionally shorten a long toe, allow for sufficient soft tissue coverage, and can avoid excessively tight closure that could compromise wound healing (see **Fig. 6**C–D). Hemostasis is largely achieved by tamponade at the time of closure. Alternately, medial and lateral flaps are used if tissue necrosis and ulceration compromises the plantar flap tissue. The patient is routinely treated with a short course of oral antibiotics, as the osteomyelitis is considered to be fully resected and is confirmed by proximal margin biopsy. The patient is allowed to weight bear in a postoperative shoe following the procedure. Sutures are typically removed at 2 to 3 weeks postoperatively depending on healing progression. The patient can then transition back into diabetic shoes and inserts as tolerated.

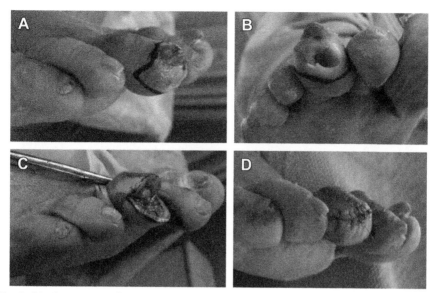

Fig. 6. (*A, B*) Lesser toe distal Syme amputation incision planning exhibiting a transverse fishmouth incision with dorsal and plantar flaps. (*C*) Postamputation with disarticulation at the distal IPJ and creation of a plantar flap. The end of the middle phalanx is removed for margin biopsy and ease of closure. (*D*) Clinical appearance following closure.

Central Toe Amputation

Central toe amputation is typically used to treat complicated neuropathic proximal IPJ and distal IPJ ulcerations, proximal spread of soft tissue infection, or osteomyelitis from tip-of-toe ulcers as well as for the resection of digital gangrene. This procedure is typically performed in the operating room unless emergent initial open amputation would otherwise be indicated in the clinical setting. Digital amputation can be performed via disarticulation at the MPJ or, alternately, retaining a portion of the base of the proximal phalanx. Preservation of the proximal phalanx base provides a spacer with the intent to minimize subsequent migration of adjacent digits. However, MPJ disarticulation may be necessary to obtain full resection of infected bone and sufficient soft tissue coverage for tension-free closure. The location of the digital ulcer, quality of digital skin, and extent of osteomyelitis therefore dictates the ideal level of amputation and soft tissue closure options. When disarticulating at the MPJ, a decision should be made regarding whether to leave articular cartilage intact versus performing resection. Although some advocate for resection of the cartilage as it is no longer perfused[15] and is at risk for subsequent necrosis,[16] others support leaving cartilage intact to act as a barrier for infection to the adjacent medullary canal.[17] We typically avoid disturbing the metatarsal head cartilage to minimize the chance of contiguous contamination and have not appreciated bacterial harboring or complications associated with poor soft tissue adherence to the joint surface. A sharp towel clamp is placed through the distal portion of the digit for ease of manipulation during dissection. The standard incision for second-digit, third-digit, and fourth-digit amputations is a vertical fishmouth incision creating medial and lateral flaps (**Fig. 7**). This incision plan allows proximal extension for access to the MPJ and metatarsal head resection if needed. If involvement of the metatarsal is suspected, a racket-type

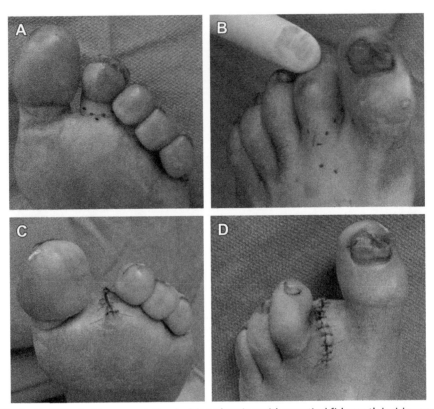

Fig. 7. (*A, B*) Central toe amputation incision planning with a vertical fishmouth incision and creation of medial and lateral flaps. (*C, D*) Clinical appearance following closure. This incision avoids the plantar weight-bearing surface but can be extended proximally to address dorsal or plantar infection or wounds.

incision can be made with the handle typically oriented along the dorsal shaft of the metatarsal to allow further inspection. If interdigital tissue quality is poor and not conducive to medial and lateral flaps, a transverse fishmouth incision with dorsal-plantar flaps can be used, but difficulty accessing the MPJ or converting to ray resection should be anticipated. This is also less desirable, as the flaps do not directly correspond with medial and lateral interdigital artery supply. An alternate approach is to create one medial or lateral digital flap opposite the interdigital ulceration that is capable of advancement and complete closure. A full-depth incision is made, with care taken to raise the flaps in a full-thickness fashion from underlying bone. Simple sutures are applied in a manner that prevents excessive skin tension and are typically left in place for 2 to 4 weeks. Deep tissue closure is not typically necessary. The patient is allowed to weight-bear in a postoperative shoe.

High-risk patients often require serial digital amputations over several years, in part because amputation has the potential to destabilize adjacent digits or make them a more exposed pressure source. In such patients who have had at least 2 digits amputated, a TMA should be considered, as it may provide a more biomechanically functional option for the patient with less chance for ulcer recurrence and subsequent amputation. Which toes remain and their condition with regard to deformity, function, and presence of pressure sores are important considerations. Functional first, second, and third toes are likely worth preserving, whereas a foot with contracted, ulcerated, and nonfunctional lesser digits may be best treated with TMA.

Central Ray Amputation

Nonhealing diabetes-related neuropathic ulcerations beneath the central metatarsal heads frequently become complicated with osteomyelitis. Ulcers in this location are oftentimes associated with transfer lesions following previous adjacent partial ray resection[18] or in the setting of a plantarflexed or elongated metatarsal. Infected metatarsal head ulcers are commonly associated with infection in the deep space of the foot. The degree of exposure and extent of incision and drainage necessary is often contingent on the severity or extent of underlying abscess. In the situation of a plantar MPJ ulceration with minimal to moderate localized purulence, the corresponding digit is amputated as previously described by using a modified vertical fishmouth incision, where the dorsal apex of the incision is extended longitudinally in full-thickness fashion to the metatarsal neck region (**Fig. 8**A–B). The plantar ulcer can be excised by extending the incision plantarly in an elliptical fashion depending on the size and depth of the ulcer. The dorsal and plantar incisions are extended proximally as needed depending on the extent of abscess and nonviable tissue. The toe is disarticulated at the MPJ. The surrounding soft tissue should be investigated for signs of abscess or extension of infection proximally through the flexor and extensor tendon sheaths. The tendons are transected and allowed to retract proximally. Careful subperiosteal dissection is performed along the medial, dorsal, and lateral metatarsal head regions with a scalpel before extending dissection onto the metatarsal neck using a McGlamry elevator. The metatarsal head is resected with a bone saw, with the cut being made behind the metaphyseal flare and beveled in a manner to prevent a prominence on the weight-bearing surface. Resection proximal to the metatarsal neck should be avoided if possible in the event a TMA would be necessary in the future. Closure is performed with nonabsorbable suture in an interrupted manner. The patient is made non weight-bearing in a postoperative shoe typically for a duration of 4 weeks or until sutures can be removed.

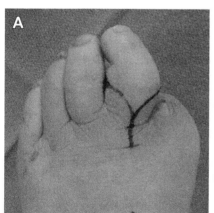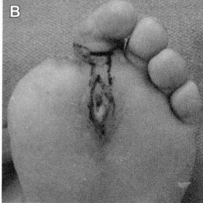

Fig. 8. (*A, B*) Standard incision planning for partial ray amputation with extension of the plantar arm for excision of plantar metatarsal head neuropathic ulceration. Alternately, dorsal and plantar flaps may be necessary in the setting of an interspace ulcer or if there is a high likelihood of converting to a TMA but should be avoided if a partial ray amputation is possible, as proximal extension of the incision is difficult.

FIFTH RAY AMPUTATION
Partial Fifth Ray Amputation

Fifth-digit amputation is often necessary for neuropathic ulcers affecting the fifth toe that are complicated by underlying osteomyelitis or gangrene. Distal Syme amputations are not typically performed in this region, as ulcerations at the tip of the fifth toe are rare. Furthermore, because of the small size of the fifth digit, complete amputation is typically necessary in terms of eradicating infection and eliminating lateral shoe pressure points. We have also observed that disarticulation at the fifth MPJ is not generally a desirable level for amputation owing to a prominent fifth metatarsal head, creating an area at risk for reulceration in the future. Consideration should be given to performing a metatarsal head resection in conjunction with fifth-digital amputation, as risk of plantar transfer lesions are lower in this region and the forefoot can be better accommodated by subsequent custom shoes and inserts. The typical partial fifth ray amputation incision would consist of a dorsal and plantar flap racquet-type incision with the handle directed proximally along the lateral aspect of the fifth metatarsal head and neck. After initial disarticulation at the fifth MPJ, the metatarsal head and neck can be dissected in full-thickness fashion. The metatarsal head is then resected immediately proximal to the metaphyseal flare. Care is taken to mildly bevel the cut to avoid plantar or lateral prominence. However, the laterally positioned racquet-type incision does not allow excision and closure of infected ulcers located beneath the fifth metatarsal head. Partial fifth ray amputation with flap closure allows for plantar fifth metatarsal head ulceration excision and closure and is essentially a mirror image of the aforementioned first ray amputation flap plan (**Fig. 9**). After full-thickness closure, the patient is typically allowed to heel weight-bear with a standard incision but remains non weight-bearing with flap closure until sutures are removed postoperatively.

Complete Fifth Ray Amputation

Depending on the extent or location of lateral column ulceration, infection, or gangrene, a complete fifth ray amputation may be necessary. This could be necessitated in the setting of recurrent ulceration and osteomyelitis after previous partial fifth ray resection. It has been our experience that resection of more than 50% of the distal fifth metatarsal shaft can lead to prominence of the residual metatarsal base stump that predisposes the patient to recurrent ulceration. If extensive resection of the fifth metatarsal beyond 50% is necessary for management of large wounds, osteomyelitis, or gangrene, a complete ray amputation should be considered. Alternately, complete fifth ray amputation may be necessary in neuropathic and decubitus pressure ulcers developing over a prominent fifth metatarsal base. Recurrent forefoot and midfoot lateral column ulcers associated with a cavus foot type or excessive inversion are commonly associated with stroke and other neuromuscular contractures. Ulcers at this location are typically large and complicated by osteomyelitis, with minimal soft tissue flexibility in the area, making them difficult to treat surgically without significant bone removal. The incision is designed to circumscribe and completely remove the ulceration in full-thickness fashion (**Fig. 10**). Dorsal and plantar soft tissue flaps are created along the lateral side of the fifth metatarsal extending out to the fifth toe. The fifth toe is circumscribed using a racquet-type incision before disarticulation at the MPJ. Subperiosteal dissection is advanced along the dorsal, lateral, and plantar aspects of the fifth metatarsal. The peroneus tertius and brevis tendons are completely detached from the base of the fifth metatarsal. A McGlamry elevator is used to free the periosteum along the medial fifth metatarsal to minimize injury to the neurovascular structures to this region. Detachment of the fifth metatarsal base is often difficult

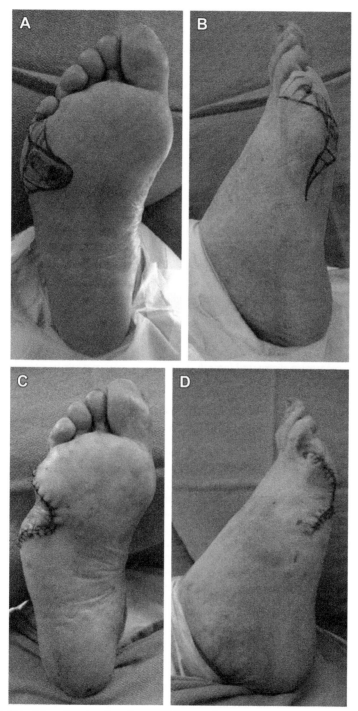

Fig. 9. (A–B) Incision planning for plantar fifth MPJ ulceration excision with partial fifth ray resection. The rotational flap is taken from the lateral forefoot extending onto the dorsal fifth digit. (C–D) This option allows for full closure of the plantar wound.

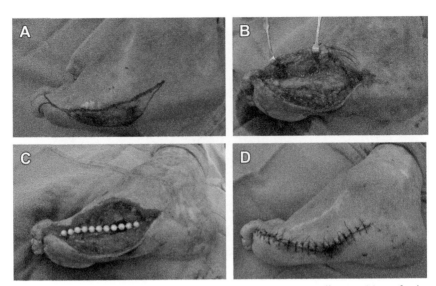

Fig. 10. (A) Complete fifth ray amputation incision planning to allow excision of a large plantar lateral ulcer. (B) The digit is disarticulated at the MTPJ and full-thickness dorsal and plantar flaps are raised along the length of the fifth metatarsal. (C–D) Immediate closure over antibiotic beads with delayed bead removal and tendon transfer is often performed.

due to robust ligamentous attachments to the adjacent cuboid and fourth metatarsal. The fifth metatarsal is distracted laterally with a towel clamp while a scalpel is used to transect soft tissue at the base of the intermetatarsal space while cutting toward the cuboid bone. The entire fifth metatarsal is then removed, with care being taken to avoid invading the fourth metatarsal or cuboid. Bone biopsy is taken from the fifth metatarsal in the area corresponding to the ulcer. The most proximal aspect of the fifth metatarsal may also be processed for clean margin biopsy. Complete fifth ray resection is typically performed in a staged approach with initial antibiotic bead application to address dead space, hematoma, and delayed tendon balancing. Once a string of antibiotic beads is placed, the dorsal and plantar flaps are closed to create a bead pouch. No drain is needed because the antibiotic beads fill the dead space, and some degree of local hematoma is desirable for maximum elution of antibiotics into the surrounding tissue. The stage 2 procedure is performed approximately 2 weeks later, with intravenous or oral antibiotics typically being given during the 2-week interval. This consists of proximal extension and opening of the wound, antibiotic bead removal, remodeling and biopsy of the cuboid, and delayed transfer of the peroneal tendons. The peroneus brevis tendon is traditionally transferred, but we prefer transfer of the peroneus longus tendon into the cuboid, as many patients with lateral midfoot ulcerations exhibit hindfoot varus[19] with a plantarflexed first ray. Detachment of the peroneus longus from the first metatarsal and medial cuneiform allows elevation of the first ray and thus partially alleviates the cavovarus deformity. This in turn decreases lateral pressure, which is desired in these circumstances. The peroneus brevis tendon can also be transferred depending on tendon quality and length or anastomosed to the transferred peroneus longus, which maximizes eversion strength. Because the distal aspect of the cuboid is prominent plantarly and laterally following fifth ray amputation, it is remodeled with a rongeur and rasp to minimize the chance of future neuropathic ulceration development in the region. The remodeled cuboid bone also provides biopsy to confirm a clean proximal margin and help direct duration of antibiotic therapy. The peroneus longus is transferred into the cuboid under anatomic tension, and soft tissue anchors can be used at the surgeon's discretion. The incision is closed in full-thickness fashion with nonabsorbable interrupted sutures, which are left in place for an additional 2 to 4 weeks, depending on healing progression. The patient remains non weight-bearing and immobilized for 6 weeks following the stage 2 procedure.[20]

TRANSMETATARSAL AMPUTATION

The TMA provides an effective and biomechanically functional treatment option in the setting of significant forefoot ulceration, infection, osteomyelitis, and gangrene.[10] Infected MPJ transfer ulcers following adjacent partial ray resection is another common situation in which TMA should be considered. Furthermore, the patient with peripheral arterial disease with insufficient blood flow to heal a more distal digital amputation despite intervention from vascular surgery or gangrene extending beyond the digital level may require a TMA. Finally, consideration should be given to the patient with previous multiple digital amputations or partial ray resection now requiring additional resection. Attempts to retain a few digits in this setting may leave multiple prominences that could predispose the patient to subsequent ulceration and repeat infection. The TMA typically provides a more definitive surgical option postoperatively. The biomechanical advantages of TMA over more proximal foot amputations are numerous. The peroneal and tibialis anterior extrinsic muscle groups maintain their insertions into the midfoot, which preserves maximal foot and ankle stability and allows for relatively normal gait from a functional standpoint. Furthermore, a long lever arm can typically be maintained with TMA to sufficiently oppose the Achilles tendon and prevent subsequent contracture. Given the relatively low possibility for contracture, as well as the presence of a reasonable metatarsal parabola, a lower likelihood of reulceration would be expected. The maintained length and low likelihood of subsequent contracture with TMA makes it a viable amputation level for accommodative orthoses and toe-box filler, which can further decrease the potential for reulceration.

The TMA may be performed under sedation with a local anesthetic block in the neuropathic patient, but general anesthesia may be needed for TMA secondary to vascular insufficiency. Incision design is based largely on the location of the wound defect and any prior ray amputation while taking into consideration the importance of preserving maximal metatarsal length.[21] The standard incision without the need to accommodate for a plantar wound defect consists of a transverse fishmouth incision with the dorsal and plantar flaps extending just distal to the MPJs. The plantar flap is often longer due to forefoot anatomy, which creates plantar-to-dorsal advancement. The medial and lateral apices typically extend to the midshaft of the first and fifth metatarsals (**Fig. 11**). In the setting of compromised arterial supply, proximal gangrene, or relatively proximal wound defect, a short TMA may be necessary with the flaps fashioned accordingly. A proximal TMA should be performed in a manner focused on preserving the first and fifth metatarsal bases in an effort to maintain extrinsic musculature attachments. Care should be taken to perform the amputation in atraumatic fashion to lower the risk for excessive blood loss, hematoma formation, and wound healing complications. Penetrating towel clamps are placed in the first and fifth digits to allow forefoot manipulation during dissection and disarticulation. The incision is made in full-thickness fashion down to bone. A plunge-cut technique is used while holding the scalpel at 90° as it is advanced transversely across the MPJs. Sharp dissection should be avoided in the intermetatarsal space until after all metatarsals have been transected with a saw to avoid violating the intermetatarsal vasculature in an attempt to limit blood loss. The dorsal flap is raised in full-thickness

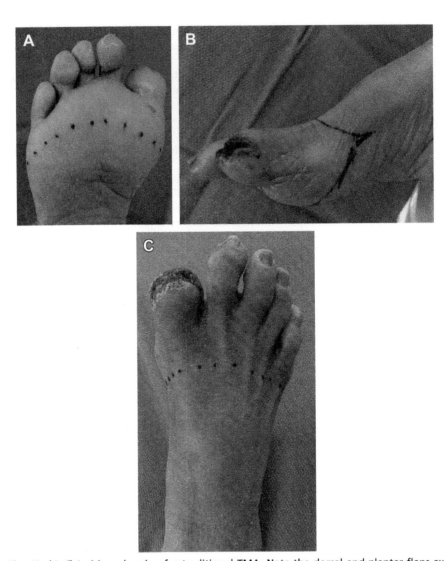

Fig. 11. (A–C) Incision planning for traditional TMA. Note the dorsal and plantar flaps extending to the level of the MPJ and the medial and lateral apices extending to the midshaft of the first and fifth metatarsals.

fashion to expose the metatarsal necks for resection. A McGlamry elevator is used to perform limited dorsal, medial, and lateral periosteal dissection at each metatarsal shaft resection site. The plantar flap is not raised but rather extended directly into the MPJs at the bases of the proximal phalanges in an attempt to minimize the likelihood of compromising the plantar flap with blind dissection. All toes are then disarticulated as a single unit and typically sent for gross analysis. The metatarsals are typically cut immediately proximal to the metaphyseal flare, with careful consideration given to maintaining a functional parabola and beveling the metatarsal cuts to avoid prominence. The metatarsal heads are then excised using careful sharp dissection. The sesamoids and plantar plate apparatus remain as part of the plantar flap until after metatarsal head excision (**Fig. 12**A–B). This allows for subsequent careful

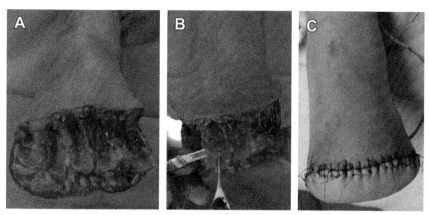

Fig. 12. (*A*) The sesamoids and individual plantar plates are left attached to the plantar flap during removal of the toes and metatarsal heads. This technique helps to ensure that the flap is full-thickness. (*B*) The plantar plates and flexor tendons are then carefully dissected off the plantar flap, which exposes the highly vascular underlying tissue and decreases the bulkiness of the flap to improve mobility. (*C*) Closure is performed with minimal touch and tension. A drain is often used to minimize hematoma risk, particularly in the setting of high-risk of bleeding.

dissection and removal to preserve the plantar flap with maximum viability and thickness. Bone biopsy is performed at the primary site of infection when appropriate. Electrocautery has not been used up to this point; the intermetatarsal arteries and other substantial vasculature are hand-tied to achieve hemostasis. During closure of the flap, some deep sutures may be placed to help decrease dead space and tension on the skin, but this is not typically necessary. Careful closure with interrupted sutures is performed with a minimal-touch technique on the skin edges (see **Fig. 12**C). When significant soft tissue defects are present following initial debridement, advanced rotational or advancement flap closure should be attempted to minimize ongoing bone exposure and large wound defects that often require a prolonged time period to heal. To achieve closure in the setting of large medial or lateral plantar wound defects, a medial or lateral plantar artery angiosome rotational flap may be necessary (**Fig. 13**). Similarly, a dorsal or plantar central wound defect may require medial and lateral flap advancement in a V-to-T fashion (**Fig. 14**). Consideration should be given to using a closed-suction drain, especially in the patient with robust vasculature or who requires some degree of perioperative anticoagulation. The drain would ideally exit on the dorsolateral or dorsomedial forefoot a couple centimeters proximal to the incision site to avoid compromising the flap or wound closure. The patient is routinely made non weight-bearing while sutures remain intact for up to 6 weeks postoperatively. Following suture removal in the office setting, the patient is fit for custom orthoses with a toe-box filler and high-top diabetic shoes to accommodate the amputation, reduce plantar foot pressure, and maximize weight-bearing functionality.[22]

MIDFOOT AND REARFOOT AMPUTATIONS

Amputations performed in the midfoot or rearfoot may be attempted as a last effort before a proximal leg amputation. Transtarsal or midtarsal (Chopart) amputations often result in contraction and instability due to the loss of extrinsic muscle attachments, creating biomechanical and prosthetic difficulties. Proximal foot amputation

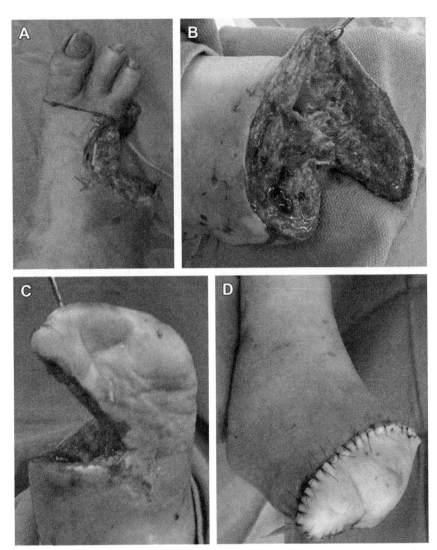

Fig. 13. (*A–D*). TMA with a medial plantar artery angiosome flap. Medial and lateral plantar artery angiosome flaps can be of utility for closure when a significant deficit is removed medially or laterally with initial debridement. A thorough understanding of angiosome principles and confirmation of arterial viability is important when considering this closure option.

is therefore typically considered only in isolated situations, such as if the patient is adamantly opposed to a proximal leg amputation. Chopart amputation is a reasonable consideration for the patient who will primarily use the limb to transfer. Many amputee candidates are beyond the age or activity level to be considered for a prosthetic leg, and maintenance of a weight-bearing extremity may significantly improve their ability to transfer independently or with minimal assistance. The elderly patient who is being considered for a second leg amputation is also a candidate for Chopart amputation if TMA is not a viable option. Younger, active, and ambulatory patients are often better served with a below-knee amputation and a functional prosthetic device.

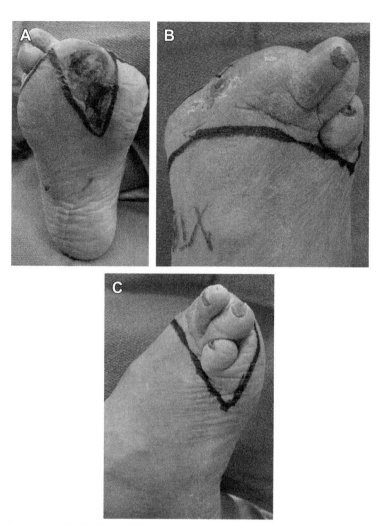

Fig. 14. (*A–C*). Modified TMA with V-to-T flap closure of large plantar wound under the central metatarsal heads. The dorsal and plantar flaps are longer compared with the traditional TMA plantar flap, nearly extending to the base of the toes. This allows adequate length after flap rotation and closure of the defect.

Tarsometatarsal joint amputation, or Lisfranc disarticulation, is a relatively viable option in the patient in whom TMA is insufficient due to extensive ulceration, osteomyelitis, or gangrene. Extrinsic musculature attachments are often compromised or lost with amputation at the tarsometatarsal joint level,[23] including the peroneus brevis and possibly the peroneus longus and tibialis anterior, depending on the resection technique. Consideration should be given to prophylactic musculotendinous balancing procedures before developing contractures, including tendo-achilles lengthening, peroneal tendon transfer into the cuboid, or posterior tibial tendon lengthening or tenotomy.

The typical incision for a Chopart amputation is a transverse fishmouth incision, with the dorsal and plantar flaps extending to the level of the tarsometatarsal joint and the medial and lateral apices extending proximally to the midtarsal joint (**Fig. 15**A–B). A

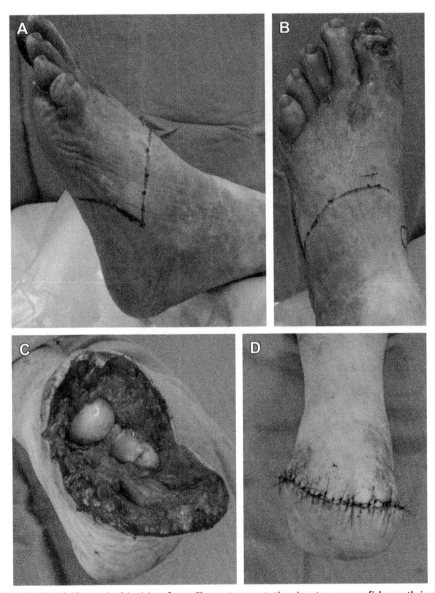

Fig. 15. (*A, B*) The typical incision for a Chopart amputation is a transverse fishmouth incision, with the dorsal and plantar flaps extending to the level of the tarsometatarsal joint and the medial and lateral apices extending proximally to the midtarsal joint. (*C*) Disarticulation is performed at the midtarsal joint before remodeling the anterior calcaneus to remove prominences. (*D*) Minimal-tension closure is performed.

larger plantar or dorsal flap may be necessary based on local vascular status or extent of nonviable tissue. The tibialis anterior and peroneus brevis tendons are carefully dissected off their midfoot attachment sites and tagged for possible subsequent transfer. Given the potential to develop a subsequent equinovarus deformity,[24,25] consideration can be given to transferring the tibialis anterior tendon onto the lateral talar neck in conjunction with tendo-achilles lengthening.[23] A full-thickness flap is raised proximally to the level of the midtarsal joint before disarticulation at the midtarsal joint (see **Fig. 15**C). The tibialis anterior tendon may be transferred into the talar neck, and the peroneus brevis tendon into the anterior calcaneus. The anterior calcaneus often requires remodeling to remove prominences that could lead to reulceration.[23] Skin is closed with a minimal-touch technique and the patient made non weight-bearing while sutures remain intact (see **Fig. 15**D).

The midtarsal joint Chopart amputation and complete foot amputation, such as the Syme amputation, have numerous disadvantages that should be considered and discussed with the patient to allow informed consent and shared decision making. Extrinsic musculature attachments are lost, which may allow the Achilles tendon to act unopposed and predispose the patient to contracture and reulceration. Tendon transfers to counteract such forces can be of limited success given the small lever arm about the ankle joint. Such disadvantages should be considered in the cohort of patients who are being considered for a midfoot or rearfoot amputation. Most patients naturally prefer to save as much of the leg as possible but do not have the insight to comprehend the positive and negative aspects of various amputation levels from a structural and functional standpoint. It is therefore the responsibility of the surgeon to properly counsel the patient before surgery regarding viable amputation options.

SUMMARY

Diabetic foot infections are a common occurrence that often require resection of nonviable bone and tissue and place the patient at risk for proximal limb loss. Many partial foot amputation options are available to assist with diabetic limb salvage when appropriate. Although a subset of diabetic patients may be better served with leg amputation for a variety of factors, most will benefit from maintaining a functional, plantigrade foot for ambulation. The first priority of surgical treatment is to effectively eradicate soft tissue infection, osteomyelitis, necrotic tissue, and gangrene to minimize potentially life-threatening systemic risks to the patient. To that end, ulceration location and the extent of osteomyelitis or necrotic tissue ultimately dictates the amputation procedure to be performed. Other procedure selection criteria are typically based on performing an amputation that maintains the most dynamic function with the least chance for ulcer recurrence in the future. A detail-oriented approach to technique is central to determining the success of lower extremity wound and amputation surgery. The techniques and pearls discussed here are important to minimizing major limb loss in the high-risk diabetic population.

REFERENCES

1. Levin ME, O'Neal LW, Bowker JH, et al. In: Levin ME, O'Neal LW, editors. The diabetic foot. 7th edition. Philadelphia: Mosby Elsevier; 2008. p. 648.
2. Oyibo SO, Jude EB, Tarawneh I, et al. The effects of ulcer size and site, patient's age, sex and type and duration of diabetes on the outcome of diabetic foot ulcer. Diabet Med 2001;18:133.
3. Ramsey SD, Newton K, Blough D, et al. Incidence, outcomes, and cost of foot ulcers in patients with diabetes. Diabetes Care 1999;22:382.
4. Singh N, Armstrong DG, Lipsky BA. Preventing foot ulcers in patients with diabetes. JAMA 2005;293:217–28.
5. Reiber GE. Epidemiology and health care costs of diabetic foot problems. In: Giurini JM, LoGerfo FW, Veves A, editors. The diabetic foot: medical and surgical management. Totowa (NJ): Humana Press; 2002. p. 39–50.

6. Aulivola B, Hile CN, Hamdan AD, et al. Major lower extremity amputation: outcome of a modern series. Arch Surg 2004;139:395–9.

7. Jones RN, Marshall WP. Does the proximity of an amputation, length of time between foot ulcer development and amputation, or glycemic control at the time of amputation affect the mortality rate of people with diabetes who undergo an amputation? Adv Skin Wound Care 2008;21:118.

8. Izumi Y, Satterfield K, Lee S, et al. Risk of reamputation in diabetic patients stratified by limb and level of amputation. Diabetes Care 2006;29:366–70.

9. Ward KH, Meyers MC. Exercise performance of lower-extremity amputees. Sports Med 1995;20:207.

10. Waters RL, Perry J, Antonelli D, et al. Energy cost of walking of amputees: the influence of level of amputation. J Bone Joint Surg Am 1976;58:42.

11. Wutschert R, Bounameaux H. Determination of amputation level in ischemic limbs: reappraisal of the measurement of TcPO2. Diabetes Care 1997;20(8): 1315–8.

12. Bacharach JM, Rooke TW, Osmundson PJ, et al. Predictive value of transcutaneous oxygen pressure and amputation success by use of supine and elevation measurements. J Vasc Surg 1992;15(3):558–63.

13. Boffeli TJ, Thompson JC. Radiation therapy for prevention of recurrent heterotopic ossification following partial metatarsal ray resection. J Foot Ankle Surg. Submitted for publication. September 2013.

14. Boffeli TJ, Peterson MC. Rotational flap closure of first and fifth metatarsal head plantar ulcers: adjunctive procedures when performing first or fifth ray amputation. J Foot Ankle Surg 2013;52:263–70.

15. Bowker JH. Partial foot amputations and disarticulations. Foot Ankle 1987;2:153.

16. Moore JC, Jolly GP. Soft tissue considerations in partial foot amputations. Clin Podiatr Med Surg 2000;17(4):631–48.

17. Rosen RC. Digital amputations. Clin Podiatr Med Surg 2005;22:343–63.

18. Gianfortune P, Pulla RJ. Sage R. Ray resections in the insensitive or dysvascular foot: a critical review. J Foot Surg 1985;24:103–7.

19. Cuttica DJ, Philbin TM. Surgery for diabetic foot infections. Foot Ankle Clin 2010; 15:465–76.

20. Boffeli TJ, Abben KW. Complete fifth ray amputation with peroneal tendon transfer—A staged surgical protocol. J Foot Ankle Surg 2012;51:696–701.

21. Wallace GF, Stapleton JJ. Transmetatarsal amputations. Clin Podiatr Med Surg 2005;22:365–84.

22. Ayyappa E. Postsurgical management of partial foot and Syme's amputation. In: Lusardi M, editor. Orthotics and prosthetics in rehabilitation. Boston: Butterworth-Heinemann; 2000. p. 379–93.

23. Decotiis JA. Lisfranc and Chopart amputations. Clin Podiatr Med Surg 2005;22: 385–93.

24. Lieberman JR, Jacobs RI, Goldstock L, et al. Chopart amputation with percutaneous heel cord lengthening. Clin Orthop 1993;296:86–91.

25. Early JS. Transmetatarsal and mid-foot amputations. Clin Orthop 1999;361: 85–90.

The Role of Plastic Surgery for Soft Tissue Coverage of the Diabetic Foot and Ankle

Peter A. Blume, DPM[a],*, Ryan Donegan, DPM[b],
Brian M. Schmidt, DPM[b]

KEYWORDS

- Wound healing • Diabetic foot and ankle • Soft tissue coverage • Wound closure
- Flaps • Skin grafts

KEY POINTS

- Diabetic foot and ankle reconstruction closure can be assisted with a thorough knowledge of flap and grafting techniques.
- Plastic surgery algorithms have been updated to include more aggressive flaps and grafting to obtain closure of defects in foot and ankle surgery.
- Be vigilant in patient selection and a thorough work-up prior to surgery will assist in obtaining optimal results.

The goal of wound healing is to obtain the best closure through the least morbid means. In the surgical treatment of the diabetic foot and ankle, the reconstructive foot and ankle surgeon is tasked with the challenge of repairing a variety of tissue defects. The decision for wound closure depends on the location of the wound and host factors (ie, tissue extensibility and the individual's healing potential). In order of increasing complexity, the clinician should consider the following reconstruction decision ladder algorithm, as set forth by Attinger and Janis.[1] According to this algorithm (**Table 1**), appropriate wound closure process should be performed by (1) performing primary closure of said wound; (2) allowing the wound to close by secondary intention, including application of various wound care products; (3) application of a negative-pressure would vacuum system; (4) skin grafting; (5) application of dermal matrices; (6) local random flaps; (7) distant flaps; (8) tissue expansion procedures; and, finally, (9) local fasciocutaneous or myofasciocutaneous flaps, island flaps, or free tissue transfers.[1-12] Wound evaluation coupled with the knowledge of various closure techniques and their indications will arm the surgeon with the tools for a successful closure.

[a] Orthopedics and Rehabilitation, and Anesthesia, Yale School of Medicine, 800 Howard Street, New Haven, CT 06519, USA; [b] Section of Podiatric Surgery, Department of Orthopedics and Rehabilitation, Yale New Haven Hospital, 20 York Street, New Haven, CT 06519, USA
* Corresponding author.
E-mail address: peter.b@snet.net

Clin Podiatr Med Surg 31 (2014) 127–150
http://dx.doi.org/10.1016/j.cpm.2013.09.006
0891-8422/14/$ – see front matter © 2014 Elsevier Inc. All rights reserved.

Table 1
New reconstructive ladder with modifications from previous model

Type of Closure	Morbidity
Free flap	Most morbid
Tissue expansion	—
Distant flaps	—
Local flaps	—
Dermal matrices	—
Skin graft	—
Negative-pressure wound therapy	—
Closure by secondary intention	—
Primary closure	Least morbid

From bottom up there is a relationship between ease and least morbid to most difficult with morbidities after previous rungs have been attempted.

Adapted from Janis JE, Kwon RK, Attinger CE. The new reconstructive ladder: modifications to the traditional model. Plast Reconstr Surg 2011;127(Suppl 1):205S–12S.

GENERAL PRINCIPLES FOR SUCCESS IN FLAPS AND GRAFTS

Planning is the most important step, and doing the planning before any incision, including an excision of the initial ulcer, is paramount. Considerations of general health, source of blood for the flap and graft, ensuring use of atraumatic technique, and minimizing the amount of undermining are critical. External factors, such as compliance, vascular status of the patient, and bony prominences, should be evaluated and never underestimated.

From a 2004 review about grafts and flaps, the success rate is well demonstrated. Using a combination of split-thickness skin grafts, local flaps, and free flaps, 56% of the patients achieved closure before discharge.[13] Even more, after performing 162 flaps in severely burned wounds of extremities, the survival rate of the flaps was 93.2%.[12] Both grafts and flaps are very viable methods to achieve closure of wounds in foot and ankle reconstruction.

PATIENT HEALTH PARAMETERS

Patients with illness complicate the workup and planning phase. Increases in many chronic diseases complicate and necessitate full history and physicals. Patients with comorbidities, such as diabetes mellitus; hypertension/hyperlipidemia; peripheral vascular disease; chronic or acute anemia; autonomic, sensory, or motor neuropathy; end-stage renal disease; active infection; history of coagulation abnormalities, including protein S deficiency; age of the patient; musculoskeletal limitations; and use of tobacco, should be addressed preoperatively and optimized.[14] Patients taking medications that affect coagulation, such as aspirin, warfarin, or heparin, must be appropriately managed. Many systemic medications, such as corticosteroids and chemotherapeutic and immunosuppressive drugs, may interfere with wound healing and this should be assessed before surgery.[15,16]

The lower extremity must be assessed for vascular and neuropathic risk factors. Positive findings of vascular insufficiency may require further consultation. The indications for vascular consultation include an ankle brachial index of less than 0.7, toe blood pressure less than 40 mm Hg, or transcutaneous oxygen tension (TcPO2) levels less than 30 mm Hg, because these measures of arterial perfusion are associated with impaired wound healing.[16] If inadequate perfusion is found, a vascular surgery consultation should be sought to determine the need for a procedure to increase perfusion.

Infections must be eliminated before flap and graft reconstruction. It is recommended to pack wounds open following infected debridement.

With respect to patient age, one classic analysis of patients undergoing nonsensate free-flap coverage of weight-bearing portions of the foot found good results in 70% of all patients. In contrast, 92% had good or excellent results in patients who were 40 years of age or younger.[17]

Finally, the patient's occupation and capacity to deal with lost time from work, including personal economy, need consideration. The patient's expectation regarding the surgical outcome, the possibility of additional surgeries, and risks, such as amputation, should be discussed.

ANATOMY

The skin envelops the entire surface of the body and consists of 2 layers: the outermost thinner layer is the epidermis and the innermost thicker layer is the dermis. The epidermis is stratified squamous epithelium arranged in distinct layers. The strata from deep to superficial are the stratum germinativum (basal layer), the stratum spinosum (prickle cell layer), the stratum granulosum, the stratum lucidum (only present on palms and soles), and the stratum corneum.[18] These strata represent different stages in the life cycle of the keratinocytes produced in the stratum basale. The keratinocytes migrate superficially to the stratum corneum and eventually slough off in approximately 19 days.[19–23]

The dermis is divided into 2 distinct layers: the superficial or papillary layer and the deep or reticular layer.[19,20,22–25] The papillary layer contains widely separated, delicate, collagenous elastic and reticular fibers enmeshed with capillaries. The papillary layer exhibits dermal papillas protruding into the epidermis. These papillae are reflected to the dermis as epidermal ridges producing finger prints. The reticular layer consists of connective tissue fibers more densely interwoven and coarser than in the papillary layer. Less dense regions produce skin tension lines. Elastin is distributed throughout the dermis. The elastin is more closely interlaced in the reticular layer.[19,20,22,23,25] Connective tissue cells, including fibroblasts, are often associated with mast cells and pigment-bearing melanophages and are distributed throughout the dermis in normal skin.

Vascularity of skin is located in the dermis and consists of a superficial (papillary) plexus and a deep (reticular) plexus. The epidermis is entirely dependent on the dermis for its blood supply. The superficial plexus branches as it enters the dermal papillae to feed the epidermis basal layer.[4,26]

Cutaneous sensation consists of Meissner corpuscles, Pacinian corpuscle receptors, root hair plexuses, and free nerve endings.[26–28] Meissner corpuscles are located in the dermal papillae and relay afferent light touch information.[28] Their location implies that they may be spared in both full-thickness skin grafts and all split-thickness skin grafts. Pacinian receptors are located in the deeper dermis or hypodermis and relay deep pressure information. Pacinian receptors are spared in full-thickness skin grafts and possibly in thick split-thickness skin grafts. Root hair plexuses relay hair motion. The hair root is in the deeper dermis and spared in full-thickness skin grafts but severed in split-thickness skin grafts. Free nerve endings are present throughout the dermis and sense painful stimuli. The free nerve endings are typically spared, resulting in pain sometimes being heightened after grafting.[23,27]

PHYSIOLOGIC CONSIDERATIONS IN FLAPS

Although it is always critical to evaluate the patient before surgery, understanding flap blood flow and the importance of surgical dissection is critical for success. Interestingly, Ian Taylor[29] described the entire body in territories that are flaps; however, his original description excluded the foot.

The most important aspect to flaps, beyond geometric principles and location, are the vascular structures at play. A random flap receives blood from a perforator artery from the dermis to the subdermis plexus. This is in contrast to an axial flap, which has a direct cutaneous artery, vein, and plexus already associated with it. By performing random flaps then, the concept of angiosomes becomes crucial for healing.

An angiosome is a composite of tissue composed of integument and underlying deep structures that is supplied or drained by a source, segmenting, or distributing artery.[29] Nomenclature of an area refers to it specific named arterial supply.[29] By having an angiosome, this allows for evaluation of a source artery for healing of a particular angiosome when planning for a flap. However, if one angiosome has succumbed to poor circulation, another angiosome may aid in perfusion of said area by use of choke vessels.

The choke vessels thereby link angiosomes and are true anastomoses that can be used to force the choke vessels to open to an area, thus allowing it to receive adequate reperfusion.[30–33] This is referred to as the delayed procedure, whereby a surgeon will raise a flap in the donor area by opening up choke vessels to the flap beyond its direct neighboring skin. Physiologically by depriving the raised flap of its normal blood supply, it increases ischemia. The ischemia forces the cells to adapt from aerobic to anaerobic metabolism that will cause a decreased pH in the vessels. When this occurs, blood vessels dilate and more blood flows to the area of interest. Secondarily, the delay technique creates a local sympathectomy, which also causes vasodilation secondary to a decrease in sympathetic tone. In summary, flaps should be positioned to maximize the vascularity of the flap.[29–31] The delay phenomenon can be appreciated clinically by demonstrating a finding in the treatment of critical limb ischemia. In those cases, if 1 of the 3 major vessels of the foot receives endovascular therapy, then wound healing is likely to be achieved.[32–34]

INTRAOPERATIVE CARE AND FLAP TECHNIQUE

Without the use of surgical delay, the surgeon must perform several steps intraoperatively to aid in flap success. For many years, flap designs were based on the concept that blood supply was from deep to superficial. However, Hidalgo and Shaw[35] proved that local plantar flaps could be designed to include sensation and blood supply without subfascial dissection. Milton[36] wrote an important article that showed the artery supply at the base of a flap determined its success and not the length-width ratio. Incision lines for the flap should be parallel to the lines of relaxed tension skin.[37] This allows minimal transverse force on them.[37] However, if concomitant bone surgery is performed, Relaxed Skin Tension Lines (RSTL) may be partially or entirely ignored.

During the surgery, atraumatic technique must be used. Skin hooks, the use of bipolar cautery, and sharp dissection must be used compared with the contrary. To raise a flap, one undermines below the subdermal plexus of the vessels in the subcutaneous plain and thus releases the tethering effect of this tissue.[38] Undermining of wound edges may help reduce tension of the flap; however, excessive undermining may endanger blood flow to the flap.[39] Also, meticulous hemostasis must be achieved before suturing.

Finally, after planning, performing, and suturing, the flap should be evaluated for excessive tension and adequate vascularity. If a flap cannot be set with 4.0 or a suture of lesser strength, then most likely there is too great of tension on the flap and delay procedure may be sensible. A variety of methods can be applied to evaluate vascularity. These include assessment of color, capillary refill timing, ultrasound Doppler examination, and even bleeding from stab wounds.[3] Best of all may be laser-assisted indocyanine green dye angiography. With adequate times spent in the OR evaluating a flap, this was shown to be a better predictor of mastectomy skin flap necrosis in breast reconstruction versus clinical judgment and fluorescein dye angiography.[40,41]

Taking these steps into consideration will aide in planning, creation, and success of a flap procedure. In the next section, a brief discussion of a few choice advancement flaps, rotational flaps, and transpositional flaps are undertaken to demonstrate their diversity for closure.

Advancement Flaps

Advancement flaps are mobile in one direction without laterality or rotation. They include single and double advancement flaps, M-plasty, T-plasty, V-to-Y, double V-to-Y, crescentic advancement flaps, and oblique sigmoid island flaps (**Table 2**). These flaps advance into the defect and are best used in a location with adequate tissue laxity and elasticity. Advancement flaps enable closure of the donor and defect site simultaneously. Advancement flaps rely on direct cutaneous perforators. As previously mentioned, care should be demonstrated to avoid excessive undermining, which may lead to flap necrosis.

Because advancement flaps do not redistribute tension, dog-ears or resulting cutaneous defects may occur (**Fig. 1**). Dog-ears can often be selectively positioned[5] and preplanning their location can reduce tension across the flap.[42] Inelastic tissue may require Biirow triangles.[42] A simple halving technique will allow closure of the flap without the use of Biirow triangles.[38]

Advancement flaps should be placed to benefit from the elasticity of the surrounding skin, while incorporating the angiosome's blood supply. Plan them perpendicular

Table 2		
List of skin flaps that can be used in foot and ankle surgery		
Advancement Flaps	**Rotation Flaps**	**Transposition Flaps**
Single or double	Single or double	Single, bi-, or modified-lobed
M Modified M-plasty	Satterfield-Jolly	Z-plasty
T	Classic	Double-Z rhomboid
V-to-Y Modified V-Y Double reverse V-Y	Catanzariti-Wehman	Double opposing Z-plasty
Double V-to-Y Crescentic advancement		Four-flap Z-plasty
Oblique sigmoid island flap		Double opposing semicircles
Y-V plasty		W-plasty Rhomboid of Limberg
V-Y-S plasty, single V-Y island flap		Flap of dufourmentel
Extended V-Y island flap		30 Transposition flap (Webster flap)
		Double or triple rhomboid
		Note flap

Listed are the different types of skin flaps that can be used to obtain closure in diabetic foot and ankle wounds. They are listed according to the motion needed to perform each flap.

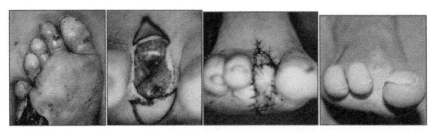

Fig. 1. Advancement Flap: Double V-Y Flap. Second digit requiring amputation (*left*), after disarticulation (*center left*), primary closure (*center right*), and end result (*right*). Note the use of V-Y flap on both dorsum and plantar surface of foot.

to the RSTL with advancement parallel to the Lines of Maximal Extensibility (LME). Although advancement flaps allow for closure of the donor and defect simultaneously, their use can be limited, due to mobility restrictions and the need for exposure to underlying osseous pathology.

Cutaneous advancement flaps, such as the T-plasty or H-plasty are commonly used to relocate standing cones away from critical structures. The "running pleated" suture technique obviates the need for large, laterally displaced Burow's triangles that are normally created during the construction of flaps such as the T-plasty and H-plasty.[43]

V-to-Y flaps

V-to-Y flaps have been used for defects in the posterior heel and ankle,[44] and on the plantar aspect of the foot.[29,45] They are also useful as an adjunct for closure of open toe amputation sites. They have been advocated for the closure of a newly formed web space during the correction of syndactyly.[46] Hand surgeons have routinely used V-to-Y flaps for digital reconstruction following traumatically amputated terminal phalanges[3] and their long-term viability has been proven. V-to-Y the direction of the LME. The width of the extended V-to-Y flap is greater than the width of the defect, because of the presence of an extension of the flap on one or both sides of the defect. If the extension is only on one side of the defect, then the length of the extension is equal to the width of the defect. If the extension is made on both sides of the defect, then the length of the extensions is equal to half the width of the defect. As the flap is advanced, the extension is hinged down into the distal aspect of the defect as a small transposition flap.

For larger defects, double V-to-Y flaps should be used.[45] Or if the necessary advancement needed to close the defect is not sufficient, then a second or even a third flap may be used.[11] If additional flaps are not available, then scrupulous dissection with the aid of loupe magnification may be performed to dissect the fibrous bands that limit motion, while sparing the perforating vessels.[11]

One of the advantages of a V-to-Y flap is that it eliminates the need for further procedures to excise dog ears or to defeat which is often necessary with direct approximation.[11] It also offsets the need for skin grafting of the donor site.

V-Y flaps suffer from design problems of the advancing edge, which is usually concave, trying to match another concave edge on the opposite side of the defect. The flap-in-flap technique uses a second V-Y flap at the advancing edge of the main flap to overcome this mismatch, and also improves the amount of advancement possible.[30]

Double V-to-Y flaps

A double V-to-Y flap, also known as a double kite flap, is useful when a defect is larger than 2 cm and may be used to close defects as large as 3 cm to 4 cm.[47] Double V-to-Y fasciocutaneous flaps have been recommended for coverage of small (up to 4 cm in diameter) lesions plantar to the metatarsal heads[45,66] and heel regions.

Double V-to-Y flaps are designed in the same fashion as the single V-to-Y flap; however, a second identical flap is designed on the opposite side of the defect. Each flap is elevated in the same manner and advanced toward each other to cover the defect.

Rotation Flaps

Rotation flaps are those that pivot about a point and move in arc motion. These flaps include single rotation flaps, double rotation flaps, and the Satterfield-Jolly. Rotation flaps provide redistribution and redirection of tension from the primary defect to the donor site.[5] They are frequently used in areas with convex surfaces or where tension lines are curved.[5] Rotation flaps can be subfascial or suprafascial as described by Hidalgo and Shaw.[35] They can also be fasciocutaneous, myocutaneous, or a combination of both. Rotation flaps can be axial or random, depending on the level of dissection and angiosome involved.

Rotation flaps can be elevated and mobilized from the non–weight-bearing arch to areas of pathologic weight-bearing surfaces. They can be used to correct defects on the plantar aspect of the heel, by including the heel pad.[48] They can also be used to cover large defects in the foot; however, they often require a skin grafting component for closure of the donor site.

Rotation flaps are an excellent adjunct in diabetic foot soft tissue coverage.[49] Because of their inherent design, they can yield a wide-based exposure to the osseous structures. Because of the required skin grafting component, strict elevation and bed rest are recommended and must be strictly enforced for 5 to 7 days, therefore increasing hospitalization and cost.

Classic rotation flap

The rotation flap consists of a triangle or 2 radians or wedges from a portion of a circle. If the rotation flap does not cover the entire defect, it may be designed larger or the length of the curved incision may be extended to free more tissue. Additionally, if even more movement is needed, a back-cut may be used to the arc of the flap. The rotation flap used to close a circular defect is usually a combination of both primary and secondary movements. The primary movement is the rotation and advancement of the flap itself over the defect and the line of the greatest tension extent from the pivot point toward the defect site. This distal tension point is the area of greatest vascular compromise. The secondary movement is the movement of the adjacent or surrounding skin in the opposite direction of the flap movement. The skin from the side of the defect opposite the flap moves over the defect more than the flap itself moves over the defect. This requires less rotation of the flap and creates less puckering at the flap pedicle. When puckers occur, they may be eliminated by cutting a Burrow triangle at the end of the incision.[50]

Single rotation flap

A single rotation flap may be used to close either a triangular defect, or circular defect (**Fig. 2**). For closure of a triangular defect, the flap is shaped semicircular in shape and rotates about a pivot point.

For a triangular defect, the base of the defect becomes part of the circumference of a semicircle. An arch-shaped flap is then designed so that the leading tip of the flap will rotate around the circumference of the circle on which the defect lies. To enable primary closure of the donor site, the flap should have a circumference five to eight times the width of the defect[54] or an area of three to four times the area of the defect.[5] The

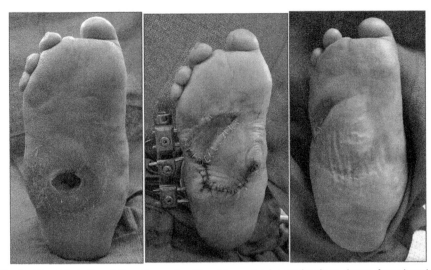

Fig. 2. Direct Rotational Flap Reconstruction: Flap raised completely and transferred at the same stage and primarily inset. A one stage reconstruction in a diabetic neuropathic patient. Pre-operatively (*Left*) and postoperatively (*right*).

major movement is in the direction of the arc of rotation of the flap. Secondary movements of the adjacent or surrounding skin in the opposite direction of the flap movement also occur. Key sutures are placed along the closing edge or shorter side of the flap. Biirow's triangles may be used at any point along the arc or longer incision, but are typically found at the base of the flap. The narrower the triangular defect, the less distance the flap will need to move,[51] and therefore, the defect should be excised with as narrow a triangle as possible.

The use of a back cut, incised at the pivot point of the flap, is controversial. Some[5,47,52] feel that the back cut allows for additional mobility of the flap, allowing it to be inset into the defect with little tension. Others feel that back cuts into the base should be avoided. If a back cut is used, it should be cut away from the base if possible or it's length should be minimized in order to avoid jeopardizing the perfusion of the flap. To avoid potentially compromising the vascularity of the flap when using a back cut, perforators into the flap should be evaluated with the use of a Doppler.[47]

If the flap will not close without excessive tension, then a maneuver described by Jackson[39] should be used. In this technique, the circumference of the rotation flap is increased, thereby lengthening the leading edge of the flap and allowing closure with decreased tension.

For a circular defect, an arc is created which is tangent to the circle, having a greater radius than the defect. The resulting flap is then rotated into the defect. In this case, there is usually a combination of both primary and secondary movements, in varying degrees depending on the elasticity of the surrounding skin. The primary movement is the rotation of the flap into the defect. The secondary movement is the movement of the surrounding tissue in the opposite direction of the flap movement. If puckering of the flap occurs, then a Biirow'striangle may need to be excised from the end of the flap.

Transposition Flaps

Transposition flaps move over adjacent intact skin to close a defect and combine the use of both rotation and advancement. These flaps include the single lobe flap, the bilobed flap, Z-plasty, double-Z rhomboid, double opposing Z-plasty, or 5-flap Z-plasty, 4-flap Z-plasty, double opposing semicircles, W-plasty, the rhomboid or Limberg flap, flap of Dufourmentel, the 30° transposition flap, double and triple rhomboid flaps, and the note flap. As with rotation flaps, these flaps redistribute and redirect tension from the primary defect to the donor site.[53] It is critical that the flap extend beyond the defect, thereby ensuring adequate length after its transposition.[42] If additional length is required, a back cut away from, or into, the base can be made, the latter option poses a risk of reducing the blood supply into the flap.[54] Transpositional flaps, like the Z-, rhomboid, and bilobed flaps, depend on pliability of adjacent skin.[55] Primary closure of the donor site is possible if the adjacent skin is elastic enough, but because of pedal skin, another skin flap or graft may be used to obtain closure.

Rhomboid or limberg flap

The rhomboid or Limberg flap is typically used to close a rhomboid-shaped defect, but may be used to close circular defects.[5,66] A flap of exactly the same shape and size as the defect, is raised and transposed 60° into the defect. While the flap covers the original defect one hundred percent, it only closes half of the total defect; the remaining defect is closed primarily.[5] The flap redistributes and redirects tension from the donor site to the recipient site, in 90°.[5]

The rhomboid flap is one of the most versatile adjuncts for closure of foot wounds and pedal defects. It can be used for correction of isolated metatarsal head lesions, with simultaneous exposure for osseous corrections such as a condylectomy, osteotomy, or metatarsal head resection. Rhomboid flaps may also be used to correct a plantar lesion. It has been adapted for dorsal lesions of the foot,[67] although greater mobility is required for primary closure. Desyndactylization procedures can also employ a rhomboid flap in the foot for plantar closure[68] or in the hand.[18]

Two parallel lines are drawn in the same direction as the LME or perpendicular to the RSTL (**Fig. 3**). These are drawn tangential to the defect. Two additional lines are drawn which complete the design of an equilateral parallelogram or rhombus with 60° and 120° angles. Four possible rhomboid flaps can then be drawn. Two of these possible rhomboid flaps will have their short axis parallel to the LME. In closing the donor site, choosing either of these two will result in the area of greatest tension to occur in the same direction as the LME.[69,70,71] if the short axis of the flap is perpendicular to the LME, the design will result in immobile flaps.[54] By using the pinch test to determine the orientation of the LME, the best flap for transposition can be chosen. Anatomical constraints or surgeon preference will result in the optimum choice from the two final possibilities.

An alternative way of viewing the design of a rhomboid flap is to first excise the lesion in the shape of a rhombus so that two of the sides are parallel to the LME. Next, extend the short diagonal of the rhombus, in either direction, by the same length as the sides of the rhombus. The final side of the flap is designed at a 60° angle to the end of the extended short diagonal and equal to the length of the sides of the rhombus. Once again, the short axis of the flap must lie parallel to the LME.

Although the complex geometry must be understood, it does not need to be strictly adhered to in order to obtain satisfactory clinical results.[5] Although the rhomboid flap was designed for use in areas where skin extensibility is significant, the flaps may be used in regions of tense skin.[72] In such cases, the entire area must be undermined, including the margins of the rhomboid defect and the base of the flap. Undermining of the donor site can be successfully achieved without compromising the surrounding subcutaneous perforators. Mobility can be increased with concomitant bone resection.

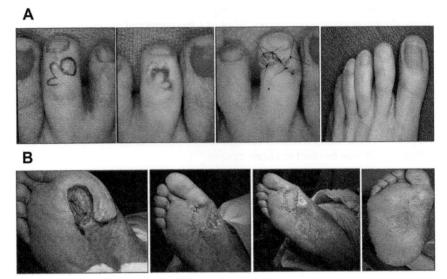

Fig. 3. (*A*) Transpositional Flap: Bilobed Flap. Second digit mucoid cyst requiring reconstruction via flap closure (*right*), following removal of cyst (center left), primary closure (*center right*), and end result (*right*). Note the size of the lobes of the prior to incision and result with closure. (*B*) Transpositional Flap: Diabetic foot ulceration closed with adjacent transposed skin from pre-operative condition (*left*) through procedure (*center left*), closure (*center right*), and end result (*right*). Note that the donor site skin received a skin graft to aid in closure.

A major advantage of the rhomboid flap is that the surgeon can choose the ideal flap from four possibilities. Another advantage is that once the length of one of the sides of the rhomboid is determined, all other incisions are the same length and calipers can be used to facilitate the design.[18] One disadvantage of the rhomboid flap is that in younger patients or when the skin is dense and thick, cosmetically significant bulges or dog ears may occur.[43]

Single lobe flap

The single lobe flap, also known as the Schrudde slide-swing plasty, may be used to close circular, oval, and semicircular defects.[56] It has been used successfully for removal of small digital lesions such as fibrous scars, intractable keratoses, and digital mucoid cysts[57] and to close a defect plantar to a metatarsal head.[35,58]

To close a circular defect, a flap in the shape of a lobe is created. The rounded end of the flap is designed with a radius smaller than the circular defect and the flap as a whole is designed to be smaller in size than the original defect. The base of the flap is placed at a 90° angle to the defect.[56]

The length to width ratio is typically 3:1.[5] Key sutures are at the distal ends of the flap. The donor region is closed primarily.

To close an oval defect, a similar flap is designed, but the base of the flap is placed at a 60° angle to the defect.[56]

The advantages of a single lobe flap are that it can be used to close a large defect, its broad base ensures good vascularity, and it avoids a secondary defect.[51] Because most lesions are circular and this flap was designed to close a circular defect, it does not involve additional excision of healthy tissue to produce a defect of a specific geometrical figure such as a rhombus.[56] It should be noted that up to one-third of the flap length may be lost during transposition of the tissue into the defect.[5]

The disadvantage of a single lobe flap may be that too much tension is created and closure is not possible without an additional lobe, in order to disperse the tension.

Bilobed flap

The bilobed flap consists of two flaps which are separated by an angle and which share a common pedicle. It was originally described by Esser[57] and later revised by Zimany.[59] It is designed to move more skin over a larger distance than is possible with a single-lobe flap and it works well in regions where skin mobility is limited.[60] It has been described as using the *Robin Hood* principle of borrowing from the *rich* laxity of a neighboring area and transposing it to a relatively *poor* area of inelastic skin.[61] This flap has been used to close defects on the plantar aspect of the foot,[62,39,59] where it is recommended for defects 1 cm to 3 cm in diameter.[39]

The bilobed flap is very versatile and can be adapted for closure of defects throughout the foot. Its uses include closure of excisions for digital cysts (**Fig. 3**A), metatarsal head ulcerations, osteomyelitis, and plantar forefoot (**Fig. 3**B) or rearfoot ulcerations, and correction of heel defects.

Since two flaps are used, two adjacent donor sites are needed to close the defect. The first lobe closes the original defect, while the second lobe closes the first flap donor site. The second flap donor site is then closed primarily. Typically the lobes are designed to be 90° from the defect and from each other, although this is not a necessity[5,62] and the angles may vary from 45° to ISO°.[59] On the plantar aspect of the foot, it is recommended that the angles be no greater than 60°.[39] The first lobe can be up to 20% smaller than the defect and the second lobe can be up to 20% smaller than the first lobe.[61] Some authors[3,8] feel that the lobes can be up to half the size of the defect they close. A general rule for lobe creation includes the following parameters. The first lobe can be 75% of the width of the original defect, while the second lobe is 50% of the original defect. The rotating base should be the only area undermined[63] although some authors recommend wide undermining.[60,61]

Some authors have found it easier and quicker to suture the second lobe into the defect caused by the first lobe and then suture the first lobe into the original defect.[64] The two apices should actually be closed first, followed by the circumferential sutures along the lobes.

An improvement in the design of bi-lobe flaps consists of rotating each lobe only 45° including a Biirow's triangle in the original design of the flap, and extending the length of the second lobe.[60] This results in a reduction of dog-ear formation, pincushioning, and distortion.[60]

The advantage of the bilobed flap is the ability to recruit large amounts of tissue by borrowing from different areas and opposing directions. The disadvantages are the length and varying directions of the incisions required.[65]

Skin Grafts

Skin grafting has a diverse role in reconstructive surgery of the foot and ankle. A graft is defined as any free tissue that is transplanted.[73] A skin graft is the separation of all or a portion of the skin from its donor site and local blood supply followed by transplantation to a recipient site.[74] The transplanted skin subsequently relies entirely on the recipient site's blood supply for survival.

Skin grafts incorporate all of the epidermis and varying depths of the dermis. A *full-thickness skin graft* consists of the epidermis and the entire dermis, whereas a *split-thickness skin graft* consists of the epidermis and a variable portion of the dermis.

According to the thickness of the dermis, split-thickness skin grafts are described as *thin, intermediate,* or *thick.* A *thin split-thickness skin graft* consists of the epidermis and approximately 0.008 to 0.012 inches of dermis. An *intermediate split-thickness skin graft* consists of epidermis and approximately 0.012 to 0.016 inches of dermis, whereas a *thick split-thickness skin graft* consists of epidermis and 0.016 to 0.020 inches of dermis.[74,75]

PHYSIOLOGY CONSIDERATIONS IN GRAFTING

It is believed that split-thickness skin grafts can reestablish circulation faster and more efficiently than full-thickness skin grafts because the harvest is more superficial in the dermis.[4,76] In split-thickness skin grafts, the number of transected vessels increases, and the number of portals available for recipient bed penetration is increased, thus revascularization of the skin graft occurs sooner.

The process of *take* of a skin graft is the revascularization and reattachment of the skin graft to the recipient site.[74] Skin grafts are a form of tissue transplantation requiring adherence and the formation of a new blood supply from the recipient bed. The 3 phases to skin graft healing are (1) the *phase of serum imbibition* (plasmatic circulation); (2) the *phase of revascularization*, a combination of neovascularization and inosculation; and (3) the *phase of organization*.[74,77–80]

The *phase of serum imbibition* is also known as plasmatic circulation because no true circulation exists between graft and recipient bed. Fibrinogen-free serum, not plasma, passively enters the graft; therefore, the phase is best termed serum imbibition.[74,81–87] At first, the graft is avascular and dependent on recipient bed fluid for nutrients. After graft placement, an effusion of clear fluid from the host bed deposits a light fibrin clot, tenuously adhering the graft to the host bed.[22,74,81,88,89] Around 24 hours and because of the graft's capillaries dilating, a fibrinogen-free suspension of erythrocytes enters the capillaries of the overlying skin. This influx of fluid into the graft causes edema over several days until venous and lymphatic circulation develop at about day 9 after graft application.[74,81,82,89] The serum imbibitions phase is not nutritional, but rather it functions to maintain graft humidity and opens the graft's vessels causing well-organized revascularization.

Serum imbibition lasts roughly 48 hours if the graft is placed on a fresh wound, but is extended if placed over an ischemic wound or shortened if the recipient site has begun proliferation. Split-thickness skin grafts may *take* well even after 4 days of ischemia, whereas full-thickness skin grafts can survive up to approximately 5 days of ischemia.[22,89] The most common complication leading to graft failure is hematoma or seroma formation within this period.

The second phase of skin graft healing is the *phase of revascularization*, which is divided into neovascularization and inosculation.[74] Neovascularization is the outgrowth of blood vessels from the recipient bed into the graft dermis at a rate of 2 mm per day. The new vessels grow into the graft from the host bed with simultaneous degeneration of the old vessels in the graft.[22,74,81,82,89] New vessel formation can occur as primary or secondary neovascularization. Blood enters the graft during this phase and the graft will gain a pink hue caused by fine extravasations on the undersurface of the graft. This signifies anastomoses are being formed. The development of vascular anastomoses with the flow of blood into the graft inhibits vascular proliferation in the recipient bed, which is a classic negative feedback mechanism.[88,89] When vascular proliferation continues uninhibited, secondary revascularization occurs.[88,89] The ischemic period is elongated during secondary revascularization and many irreversible degenerative processes occur within the graft. When inhibition of vascular growth is absent, the capillaries grow into the graft in a manner that differs from normal skin. The graft heals with a smooth, tight, and silvery shine on its surface. In larger grafts, it is common for both types of revascularization to exist.[79,80] Inosculation occurs where circulation is restored in the original graft vessels through anastomoses with the recipient bed vessels.[22,74,88,89] A predominance of new capillary channels within the graft dermis suggests an active neovascularization process.[22,74,88,89]

The *phase of organization* begins when the graft has fully adhered to the recipient bed.[51] The graft now functions in a similar manner to native peripheral skin. The graft match and durability is a function of the percentage of dermis transplanted. This phase begins with adherence of the graft to the host, whereas the recipient bed produces exudate containing plasma, erythrocytes, and leukocytes.[22,88,89] The fibrinogen in the exudate precipitates into fibrin that allows for graft adherence to the host bed. The succeeding fibrinogen-free serum penetrates the fibrin layer and enters the graft dermis to provide nourishment and assists in maintaining a moist environment until a more thorough blood supply can be established.[86] Leukocytes enter the dermis and eventually focus on degenerating appendages and epidermis.[22,86,88,89] Leukocytes will remain until reestablishment of circulation is complete. Fibroblasts and leukocytes penetrate the fibrin layer from day 4 to day 8 as the fibrin clot is resorbed and reorganized. By day 9, fibroblasts have fastened the graft to the recipient bed's reticular layer of the dermis.

Throughout the first 25 to 30 days after graft application, the graft nerves degenerate.[27,89,90] At approximately 2 months, reinnervation begins, with pain sensation returning first, followed by touch, hot and cold distinction, and finally the ability to perspire.[27,91,92] This process can occur for as long as 2 years. Graft reinnervation is best in full-thickness skin grafts and less in thin split-thickness skin grafts; however, the rate at which sensation returns is quickest in thin split-thickness skin grafts and slowest in full-thickness skin grafts.[27] In all types of sensation, the graft tends to assume the sensory pattern of the recipient bed.[27,91] Grafts placed over periosteum or muscle develop poor sensation.[27] Placement of the graft nerve fibers parallel to the direction of the ingrowing nerves does not appear to affect the speed or quality of reinnervation.[27] The application of several small grafts versus one large graft can adversely affect the reinnervation process.[27,91]

SKIN CONTRACTION IN SKIN GRAFTS

Two types of skin contraction occur with skin grafting. Primary contraction occurs at the graft site where graft is removed from the donor site. Contraction occurs greater in full-thickness skin grafts than in split-thickness skin grafts, likely from the elastin fibers in the dermis.[74,76,93–95] Full-thickness skin grafts retract approximately 44%, intermediate split-thickness skin grafts retract approximately 22%, and thin split-thickness skin grafts retract approximately 9%.[88,96,97] Tension applied to the graft when applied recipient bed reestablishes graft length and width.

Secondary contraction occurs once the graft is fixed to the recipient bed.[95] Secondary contraction results from the host bed myofibroblasts within the wound pulling the skin graft. Full-thickness skin grafts are more resistant to secondary contraction than split-thickness skin grafts.[98] The greater the percentage of dermis in the graft, the less the skin graft contracts secondarily. Initial invasion of myofibroblasts is equal in full-thickness skin grafts, split-thickness skin grafts, and in granulating wounds.[98] It has been observed that the myofibroblast life cycle is much shorter in full-thickness skin grafts as compared with split-thickness skin grafts; therefore, the greater the relative thickness of graft dermis, the speedier the myofibroblast life cycle.[95] Relative thickness refers to the percentage of dermis in the graft. In addition to the shorter myofibroblast life cycle, the enzyme prolyl hydroxylase necessary for collagen synthesis is inhibited to a greater degree in full-thickness skin grafts compared with split-thickness grafts; thus, full-thickness skin grafts resist secondary contraction better than thin split-thickness skin grafts.[22,76,88,89,93,99]

INDICATIONS

Many indications exists for skin grafting in foot and ankle surgery. Sterile ulcerations/burns, traumatic soft tissue loss, defects from flap donor sites, tumor resections, defects from incisional drainage, and desyndactylization are some indications for grafts in the lower extremity.[86,100–106]

PREOPERATIVE PREPARATION OF THE RECIPIENT BED

Recipient bed preparation is a vital component of skin grafting. The bacterial count should be less than 10^5 organisms per gram of granulation tissue.[107–110] A recipient wound bed ready for skin grafting should have a red hearty granular base with increased skin lines and neoepithelialization at the wound edges.[98] Periwound erythema should be absent. Wound conversion from chronic to acute is paramount to a successful take.[76,93,107,108,111]

Wound debridement is accomplished with the following techniques: (1) topical treatment, (2) serial debridement, and (3) trial porcine skin grafting or use of another biologic wound dressing.[1,8] Topical treatment with silver sulfadiazine 3 times a day after serial debridements will often decrease the bacterial count. Silver sulfadiazine may actually stimulate epithelialization.[112–115] Other agents, such as 3% hydrogen peroxide, 1% povidone iodine, 0.25% acetic acid, and 0.5% hypochlorite are acceptable as a one-time use to decrease bacterial load. These agents can be used daily but care is needed because of their cytotoxic effects on epithelial migration at higher concentrations.[88] Less potent concentrations of these agents are not toxic and may render them nonantibacterial.[116]

Porcine xenografting can be helpful in determining the potential viability of a split-thickness skin graft. Advantages of xenografts include the lack of donor site morbidity. The recipient bed is prewounded, which allows for conversion to the proliferative phase, which may decrease time to graft take when the permanent graft is applied.[1,75] Porcine grafts can be used to clean a wound unless the wound is infected with gram-negative bacteria.[117] Gram-negative bacteria thrive in the porcine graft and the wound actually worsens. If the porcine graft shows signs of take by day 7 to 10, then the wound is clean enough to accept the autograft.[76,98]

INTRAOPERATIVE PREPARATION OF THE RECIPIENT BED

Skin graft failure is often a result of inappropriate preparation of the recipient bed; therefore, careful attention is placed on debridement techniques. Intraoperative preparation of the recipient bed begins with excision of the wound edges and curettage of the granulation tissue from the base of the wound to create a clean, healthy bed for skin graft application. Granulation tissue has many crevices that allow for bacterial colonization.[118] The wound bed is then pulse lavaged with plentiful amounts of saline or lactated Ringers. The fluid velocity and quantity that is used for lavaging, called detergent action, allows for cleansing of the wound. Antibiotic-containing fluids are not necessary in the pulse-lavage. Once the irrigation is complete, gloves, gowns, and light handles need to be changed to maintain sterility. The surgical site is re-draped and a separate sterile closure table used for the remainder of the procedure.

TECHNIQUE OF SPLIT-THICKNESS SKIN GRAFT DONOR SITE HARVESTING WITH POWER INSTRUMENTATION

The donor site should be chosen and measured preoperatively, allowing the patient to be properly positioned for the harvest. The donor region is shaved preoperatively and prepped in the usual aseptic manner. General, spinal, or local anesthesia can be used. The donor site can be infiltrated with local anesthesia with or without epinephrine.[114,119]

Povidone-iodine is regularly used to prep the donor site, but should be washed off before harvesting. The povidone-iodine causes the dermatome to stick to the skin and can cause the operator to "skip," quite possibly increasing the need for more skin to be harvested. Zimmer now recommends using sterile saline while harvesting the skin graft to increase the life of the instruments.

Before initiating the graft harvest, the dermatome thickness can be checked at 0.015 inch by introducing a no. 15 Bard-Parker scalpel blade between the cutting blade and the base. The dermatome blade can be dulled with continuous passes of the no. 15 blade between the dermatome blade and base.[22,76,93]

The graft harvesting requires the dermatome, with power running, to be set flat on the skin. The dermatome is advanced on the skin surface with constant pressure. It is useful to visualize the dermatome as an airplane landing on an aircraft carrier, moving along the runway, and taking off again. Having an assistant apply pressure to the skin in front of the dermatome with fingers can ease the process by creating uniform tension during removal, resulting in a more accurate cut. Another assistant can then grasp the skin, with atraumatic pickups, to allow the graft thickness to be judged. Thicker grafts are opaque and thinner grafts are translucent.

Once harvested, the graft is placed on a sterile saline-soaked sponge until use. The graft can be meshed or pie-crusted. If donor site bleeding is uncontrolled, the site may be sprayed with topical thrombin or 1:200,000 dilute epinephrine. Intraoperatively, the site may be temporarily covered with saline-soaked gauze or a sheet of Xeroform (Sherwood Medical Industries, St Paul, MN).

MESHING AND PIE-CRUSTING

A split-thickness skin graft can be used whole, meshed, or pie crusted.[120] The technique of meshing involves placing the graft on a plastic carrier and hand-cranking the tissue through the meshing machine.[121–124] Meshed grafts should not exceed a ratio of 1.5 to 1.0. A ratio greater than 1.5 to 1.0 leaves a crisscross pattern on the skin because of the inability of the larger spaces to fill in by epithelial migration from the surrounding graft. Another reason not to overexpand the mesh graft is that it allows the recipient bed to contract more than smaller meshed grafts. Meshing has 3 distinct advantages. First, it allows for expansion of the skin graft to cover larger areas. Second, it adheres better to irregular surfaces. Third, it allows excessive fluid to drain from the recipient bed and thereby reduces the risk of hematoma/seroma formation below the graft.[22,76,93]

Pie-crusting is the practice of placing the split-thickness onto a hard surface, dermis side up, and using a scalpel to create a variable number of small cuts or slits into the graft.[124,125] Pie crusting, like meshing, allows for drainage, decreasing the likelihood of hematoma or seroma formation beneath the graft. Pie crusting does not have the crisscross pattern in the healed skin like meshed skin grafts, but has the disadvantage of not allowing the same degree of subgraft hematoma or seroma drainage or expansion.

APPLICATION OF THE SPLIT-THICKNESS SKIN GRAFT

Split-thickness skin grafts, especially if meshed, have a tendency to fold on themselves. Patience and a steady hand are required for insetting the graft. Either the meshing plate, saline-soaked gauze, or Telfa (Kendall Co, Boston, MA) and pickups, are used to transport the graft onto the recipient bed. There are 4 ways to adhere the graft to the recipient site: (1) skin staples; (2) simple interrupted suture technique with 4.0 or 5.0 monofilament nylon; (3) running 5.0 polyglycolic acid, polyglactin, chromic, or plain gut stitch; and (4) nothing at all.[190] It is not advisable to stretch the graft or to let it fold back on itself. The surgeon may spray the recipient bed with topical thrombin to aid in graft adherence. Finally, once in place, trimming of the excess skin graft is completed for appropriate fit.[190]

DRESSING THE SKIN GRAFT

Once the graft is in place on the recipient bed, the graft should be covered with saline-soaked cotton balls and Xeroform (Sherwood Medical Industries) placed directly on the graft. This stent or bolster dressing applies pressure to the graft over the recipient bed, preventing hematoma and seroma formation beneath the graft and reducing mechanical shear forces by adhering the graft over irregular surfaces.

As for the skin graft itself, numerous theories have been practiced to aid in graft take. Most common is the bolstered dressing, but more recently the combination of wound vacuum-assisted closure has greatly improved skin graft take, and lessened seroma and hematoma formation.[126,127] Once prewounding, whether done with debridement or synthetic skin graft placement, like Integra (Integra LifeSciences, Plainsboro, NJ), is complete, the Split Thickness Skin Graft (STSG) is taken and applied to the wound. Following this, a wound vacuum is placed on the area for 5 days. During this period of time, the wound vacuum is not changed unless complications arise. The vacuum will reduce shearing forces and eliminate most fluid build up between the graft and bed to allow for serum imbibition.[128,129] It is also ideal to have the patient remain non–weight-bearing during this time period because of risk of disconnecting the vacuum and allowing excess fluid to build up.

After 5 days is complete, the vacuum is removed. In a small study, Hegelson and colleagues[130] demonstrated that with appropriate prewounding and STSG placement associated with wound vacuum closure, closure was obtained in more than 90% of their patients. Even more, is that with the use of the wound vacuum after STSG placement, the amount of skin graft lost reduces length of hospitalization.[131]

A Cochrane database review agrees that loss of skin graft is less in NPWT–STSG groups, but it is suggested that hospital-based products to create an Negative Pressure Wound Therapy (NPWT) atmosphere are equivalent to the available commercial-based products, and economics may be of concern for optimal results. It is also suggested that more high-powered data need to be presented before final conclusions can be made.[132]

POSTOPERATIVE CARE

Postoperative care of the limb is critical to the prevention of potential complications. The extremity is placed on strict elevation and non–weight-bearing status for 5 days to allow development of graft-host circulation. A sequential dangling regimen is undertaken consisting of 5 minutes per hour on day 7, 10 minutes per hour on day 8, and 15 minutes per hour on day 9, which allows the skin graft to adjust to venous gravitational force without heightened edema.[22,76,88,93] Physical therapy begins near the third postoperative week to increase range of motion. By 4 to 6 weeks postoperatively, the patient may progress to guarded weight bearing with an appropriate assistance device. The foot should remain wrapped with an ACE bandage whenever it is in a dependent position. By 6 to 8 weeks postoperatively, the patient may progress to full weight bearing with decreasing assistance as tolerated. Preoperative physical therapy and gait training is often beneficial.

SKIN GRAFT AND SKIN FLAP COMPLICATIONS

Many factors may cause skin graft and flap failure. Complications include infection, mechanical shearing forces, inadequate vascularity, seroma and hematoma formation, and technical/surgical error.[4,22,88]

Infection is another cause of that leads to failure of reconstruction closure attempts. Sterilization of the recipient bed before surgery placement is necessary. Organisms including *Staphylococcus aureus, Pseudomonas*, and *beta-hemolytic Streptococcus* have been identified in graft failure more than other organisms.[109,133] To demonstrate this, a study from 1998 revealed both a 35% and 25% decrease in graft take in grafts infected with *S aureus* and *Pseudomonas*, respectively.[134]

Inadequate vascularity can be avoided by proper patient selection elicited through an History and Physical (H&P) and noninvasive vascular examinations as needed.[14,135,136] If the patient has peripheral vascular disease, then working as a team with a vascular surgeon is crucial.[32] Intrinsically, vascular failure can result from flap design and geometric parameters or, extrinsically, due to venous and arterial issues as mentioned previously. Many times, patients with decreased perfusion will need a bypass graft to reperfuse the affected area before podiatric intervention.[32,33]

The commonest complication of skin grafts is hematoma formation. It prevents graft recipient bed contact increasing the ischemic period and decreasing the chance of graft survival.[76,116] If there is 0.5 mm of fluid between the graft and the recipient bed, then revascularization is delayed 12 hours. If the amount of fluid is increased to 5.0 mm, then revascularization is delayed by 5 days if the graft survives at all.[76] The best way to prevent hematoma formation from the beginning is to achieve hemostasis. If excessive bleeding is noted, the team may want to delay graft placement by 24 hours. Seroma occur where lymphatic channels meet, as in the groin region.[22,88,89] In split-thickness skin grafts, elevation by seroma may not permit epithelialization on the underside of the graft, thereby inhibiting revascularization that can result in sloughing of the graft and/or graft failure.

Long-term mechanical and pressure distribution issues should be addressed before surgery. Skin grafts should be avoided on weight-bearing surfaces.[124,137–139] Consider that skin grafting normally occurs in patients who do not have "normal" feet and will therefore unlikely have normal plantar pressure distribution. Many patients have had previous foot reconstruction, creating mechanical and structural instability, or have markedly deformed feet.[137,140]

Intraoperatively, the use of nontraumatic techniques can doom sensitive surgery. As mentioned previously, excessive undermining and lack of attention to details, such as not making an incision perpendicular to skin, will decrease the chances of success. The inexperienced surgeon may and can do harm without careful planning and execution of said plan.

After surgery, there are other factors that can lead to surgical site failure. External healing confounders, such as cigarette smoking, uncontrolled diabetes mellitus, unrecognized malnutrition, or use of medications that result in vitamin deficiencies, also increase the risk of failure.[6,141,142] Patient noncompliance, poor dressing technique, and irregular follow-up can also complicate the postoperative course of these surgeries. Healing is often a long course that involved many ups and downs. Be open and be vigilant with patient care after flap and graft surgery because pain, infection, and delayed healing may be encountered and can be difficult to resolve.

REFERENCES

1. Janis JE, Kwon RK, Attinger CE. The new reconstructive ladder: modifications to the traditional model. Plast Reconstr Surg 2011;127(Suppl 1):205S–12S.
2. Stedman's medical dictionary. 28th edition. Baltimore (MD): Lippincott Williams & Wilkins; 2005.
3. Attinger C. Soft-tissue coverage for lower-extremity trauma. Orthop Clin North Am 1995;26(2):295–334.
4. Attinger CE. Use of soft tissue techniques for salvage of the diabetic foot. In: Kominsky S, editor. Medical and surgical management of the diabetic foot. St Louis (MO): Mosby; 1994. p. 323–66.
5. Hirshowitz B, Mahler D. T-plasty technique for excisions in the face. Plast Reconstr Surg 1966;37(5):453–8.
6. Hirshowitz B, Karev A, Levy Y. A 5-flap procedure for axillary webs leaving the apex intact. Br J Plast Surg 1977;30:48–51.
7. Larrabee WF. Bilobed flap reconstruction of the temporal forehead. Arch Otolaryngol Head Neck Surg 1992;117:983–4.
8. Attinger CE, Bulan EJ. Debridement: the key initial first step in wound healing. Foot Ankle Clin 2001;6(4):627–60.
9. Sumpio BE, Blume PA. Contemporary management of foot ulcers. In: Pierce WH, Matsumura JS, Yao JS, editors. Trends in vascular surgery. Chicago: Precept Press; 2002. p. 277–90.
10. Marcinko DE. Plastic surgery in podiatry (simplified illustrated techniques). J Foot Surg 1988;27(2):103–10.
11. Satterfield VK, Jolly GP. A new method of excision of painful planter forefoot lesions using a rotation advancement flap. J Foot Ankle Surg 1994;33(2):129–34.
12. Huang SR, Li XY, Wang H, et al. The use of local flap in repairing deeply burned wound of extremities. Zhonghua Wai Ke Za Zhi 2005;43(3):182–4 [in Chinese].
13. Baumeister S, Dragu A, Jester A, et al. The role of plastic and reconstructive surgery within an interdisciplinary treatment concept for diabetic ulcers of the foot. Dtsch Med Wochenschr 2004;129(13):676–80.
14. Ratner D. Skin grafting: from here to there. Dermatol Clin 1998;16:75–90.
15. Wang AS, Armstrong EJ, Armstrong AW. Corticosteroids and wound healing: clinical considerations in the perioperative period. Am J Surg 2013;206:410–7.
16. Imanishi N, Kish K, Chang H, et al. Anatomical study of cutaneous venous flow of the sole. Plast Reconstr Surg 2007;120(7):1906–10.
17. Hale DS, Dockery GL. Giant keratoacanthoma of the planter foot: a report of two cases. J Foot Ankle Surg 1993;32(l):75–84.
18. Sumpio BE, Paszkowiak JJ, Blume PA. Vascular ulcers. In: Creager J, Olin J, editors. Vascular medicine. St Louis (MO): Mosby; 2006. p. 880–93.
19. Dockery GL. Anatomy of the skin. In: Bralow L, editor. Cutaneous disorders of the lower extremity. Philadelphia: WB Saunders Co; 1997. p. 1–8.

20. Marieb EN. The integumentary system. In: Marieb EN, editor. Human anatomy and physiology. New York: The Benjamin/Cummings Publishing Co, Inc; 1991. p. 138–54.

21. Muhart M, McFalls S, Kirsner RS. Behavior of tissue-engineered skin: a comparison of a living skin equivalent, autograft, and occlusive dressing in human donor sites. Arch Dermatol 1999;135:913–8.

22. Rudolph R, Ballantyne DL. Skin grafts. In: McCarthy JH, editor. Plastic surgery. Philadelphia: W.B. Saunders Company; 1990. p. 2221–74.

23. McLafferty E, Hendry C, Alistair F. The integumentary system: anatomy, physiology and function of skin. Nurs Stand 2012;27(3):35–42.

24. Bennett RG. Cutaneous structure, function, and repair. In: Bennett RG, editor. Fundamentals of cutaneous surgery. St Louis (MO): Mosby; 1988. p. 17–99, 274–309.

25. Bloom W, Fawcett DW. Epithelium and glands and secretion. In: Fawcett DW, editor. A textbook of histology. New York: Chapman and Hall; 1994. p. 57–107.

26. McGrath JA, Eady RA, Pope FM. Rook's textbook of dermatology. 7th edition. Hoboken, New Jersey: Blackwell Publishing; 2004.

27. Pontn B. Grafted skin: observations on innervation and other qualities. Acta Chir Scand 1960;(Suppl 257):1–78.

28. Wada H, Mihara K. Nerve endings in palm skin grafts. Ann Plast Surg 1989;22:461–6.

29. Taylor GI, Palmer JH, McManamny D. The vascular territories of the body (angiosomes) and their clinical applications. In: McCarthy JG, editor. Plastic surgery. Philadelphia: W.B. Saunders Company; 1990. p. 329–78.

30. Taylor GI, Corlett RJ, Caddy CM, et al. An anatomic review of the delay phenomenon: II. Clinical applications. Plast Reconstr Surg 1992;89(3):408–16.

31. Callegari PR, Taylor GI, Caddy CM, et al. An anatomic review of the delay phenomenon: I. Experimental studies. Plast Reconstr Surg 1992;89(3):397–407.

32. Alexandrescu V, Söderström M, Venermo M. Angiosome theory: fact or fiction? Scand J Surg 2012;101(2):125–31.

33. Osawa S, Terashi H, Tsuji Y, et al. Importance of the six angiosomes concept through arterial-arterial connections in CLI. Int Angiol 2013;32(4):375–85.

34. Ino K, Kiyokawa K, Akaiwa K, et al. A team approach to the management of intractable leg ulcers. Ann Vasc Dis 2013;6(1):39–45.

35. Hidalgo DA, Shaw WW. Anatomic basis of plantar flap design. Plast Reconstr Surg 1986;78(5):627–36.

36. Milton SH. Pedicled skin flaps: the fallacy of the length-width ratio. Br J Surg 1961;57:502.

37. Jackson IT, editor. Local flaps in head and neck reconstruction. New York: The CV Mosby Company; 1985. p. 6–33.

38. Lesavoy MA. Local incisions and flap coverage. In: McCarthy JG, editor. Plastic surgery. Philadelphia: W.B. Saunders Company; 1990. p. 4441–58.

39. McCarthy JG. Introduction to plastic surgery. In: McCarthy JG, editor. Plastic surgery. Philadelphia: W.B. Saunders Company; 1990. p. 55–68.

40. Phillips BT, Lanier ST, Conkling N, et al. Intraoperative perfusion techniques can accurately predict mastectomy skin flap necrosis in breast reconstruction: results of a prospective trial. Plast Reconstr Surg 2012;129(5): 778e–88e.

41. Pattani KM, Byrne P, Boahene K, et al. What makes a good flap go bad? A critical analysis of the literature of intraoperative factors related to free flap failure. Laryngoscope 2010;120(4):717–23.

42. Elliot RA. Rotation flaps of the nose. Plast Reconstr Surg 1969;44(2):147–9.

43. Rooks MD. Coverage problems of the foot and ankle. Orthop Clin North Am 1989;20(4):723–36.
44. Blume PA, Moore JC, Novicki DC. Digital mucoid cyst excision by using the bilobed flap technique and arthroplastic resection. J Foot Ankle Surg 2005; 44(1):44–8.
45. Cuono CB. Double Z-plasty repair o f large and small rhombic defects: the double-Z rhomboid. Plast Reconstr Surg 1983;71(5):658–67.
46. Ono I, Gunji H, Sato M, et al. Use of the oblique island flap in excision of small facial tumors. Plast Reconstr Surg 1993;91(7):1245–51.
47. Attinger C, Cooper P, Blume P. Vascular anatomy of the foot and ankle. In: Jurkiewicz MJ, Culbertson JH, editors. Operative techniques in plastic and reconstructive surgery. Los Angeles: General Publishing Group; 1996. p. 183–98.
48. Hirshowitz F, Kaufman T, Amir I. Biwinged excision for closure of rounded defect. Ann Plast Surg 1980;5:372–80.
49. Boffeli TJ, Peterson MC. Rotational flap closure of first and fifth metatarsal head plantar ulcers: adjunctive procedure when performing first or fifth ray amputation. J Foot Ankle Surg 2013;52(2):263–70.
50. Shaw WW, Hidalgo DA. Anatomic basis of plantar flap design: clinical applications. Plast Reconstr Surg 1986;78(5):637–49.
51. Esser JFS. estieltelokaleNasenplastikmitZweizipfligemlappenDeckung des SekundarenDetektesvomerstenZipfeldurch den Zweiten. Dtsch Z Chirurgie 1918; 143:385.
52. Keser A, Sensoz O, Mengi AS. Double opposing semicircular flap: a modificationof opposing Z-plasty for closing circular defects. PlastReconstrSurg 1998; 102(4):1001–7.
53. Jackson IT. Local flaps in head and neck reconstruction. New York: Mosby; 1985. p. 6–33.
54. Dockery GL, Christensen JC. Principles and descriptions of design of skin flaps for use on the lower extremity. Clin Podiatr Med Surg 1986;3(3):563–77.
55. Chasmar LR. The versatile rhomboid (Limberg) flap. Can J Plast Surg 2007; 15(2):67–71.
56. Morain WD, Dellon AL, MacKinnon SE, et al. Current concepts in plastic surgery for the diabetic. Adv Plast Reconstr Surg 1987;4:1–36.
57. Gidumal R, Carl A, Evanski P, et al. Functional evaluation of nonsensate free flap to the sole o f the foot. Foot Ankle 1986;7(2):118–23.
58. Brobyn TJ, Cramer LM, Hulnick SJ. Facial resurfacing with the Limberg Flap. Clin Plast Surg 1976;3(3):481–90.
59. Sanchez-Conejo-Mir J, Bueno Montes J, Moreno Gimenez JC, et al. The bilobed flap in sole surgery. J Dermatol Surg Oncol 1985;11(9):913–7.
60. Sarrafian SK. Anatomy of the foot and ankle. 2nd edition. Philadelphia: JB Lippincott; 1993. p. 329.
61. Park S, Eguchi T, Tokioka K, et al. Reconstruction of incomplete syndactyly of the toes using both dorsal and plantar flaps. Plast Reconstr Surg 1996;98(3): 534–7.
62. Attinger C, Bulan EJ, Blume PA. Pharmacological and mechanical management of wounds. In: Mathes SJ, editor. Plastic surgery, vol. 1. St. Louis: Elsevier; 2006. p. 863–99.
63. Fleetwood FR, Barret SL, Day SV. The burrow advancement flap for closure of plantar defects. J Am Podiatr Med Assoc 1987;77(5):246–9.
64. Gillies H, Millard DR Jr. In: Gillies HD, Millard DR Jr, editors. The principles and art of plastic surgery. Boston: Little, Brown; 1957. p. 5.

65. Lister GD, Gibson T. Closure of rhomboid skin defects: the flaps of Limberg and Dufourmentel. Br J Plast Surg 1972;25:300–14.
66. Lombardo M, Aquino JM. Local flaps for resurfacing foot defects: a vascular perspective. J Foot Surg 1982;21(4):302–4.
67. Becker H. The rhomboid-to-W technique for excision of some skin lesions and closure. Plast Reconstr Surg 1979;64(4):444–7.
68. Bosch E, Kreitner KF, Peirano MF, et al. Safety and efficacy of gadofosvesetenhanced MR angiography for evaluation of pedal arterial disease: multicenter comparative phase 3 study. AJR AmJ Roentgenol 2008;190(1):179–86.
69. Borges AF. The W-plastic versus the Z-plastic scar revision. Plast Reconstr Surg 1969;44(1):58–62.
70. Bouche RT, Christensen JC, Hale DS. Unilobed and bilobed skin flaps. Detailed surgical technique for plantar lesions. J Am Podiatr Med Assoc 1995;85(1):41–8.
71. Chang TJ, Stanifer EG, Jimenez AL. Plastic repair techniques: skin plasties and local flaps. In: Tucker GA, editor. Reconstructive surgery of the foot and leg'93. Tucker, GA: Podiatry Institute Publishing; 1993. p. 52–65.
72. Stedman's medical dictionary. 26th edition. Baltimore: Lippincott Williams & Wilkins; 1995. p. 660.
73. Angel MF, Giesswein P, Hawner P. Skin grafting. In: Evans GRD, editor. Operative plastic surgery. New York City, New York: McGraw-Hill; 2000. p. 59–65.
74. Barratt GE, Koopmann CF. Skin grafts: physiology and clinical considerations. Otolaryngol Clin North Am 1984;17:335–51.
75. Kirsner RS, Eaglstein WH, Kerdel FA. Split-thickness skin grafting for lower extremity ulcerations. Dermatol Surg 1997;23:85–91.
76. Attinger CE. Plastic surgery techniques for foot and ankle surgery. In: Myerson JW, editor. Foot and ankle disorders. Philadelphia: W.B. Saunders; 2000. p. 585–684.
77. Converse JM, Uhlschmid GK, Ballantyne DL. Plasmatic circulation in skin grafts. Plast Reconstr Surg 1969;43:495–9.
78. Mast BA. Healing in other tissues. Surg Clin North Am 1997;77:529–47.
79. Mathes SJ. Reconstructive surgery: principles, anatomy and techniques. New York: Elsevier Science; 1997.
80. Serafin D. Atlas of microsurgical composite tissue transplantation. New York: Elsevier Science; 1996.
81. Clemmesen T. The early circulation in split skin grafts. Acta Chir Scand 1962;124:11.
82. Clemmesen T. Experimental studies on the healing of free skin autografts. Dan Med Bull 1967;14(Suppl 2).
83. Converse JM, Ballantyne DL, Rogers BO, et al. A study of viable and non-viable skin grafts transplanted to the chorio-allontoic membrane of the chick embryo. Transplant Bull 1958;5:108.
84. Converse JM, Filler M, Ballantyne DL. Vascularization of split-thickness skin autografts in the rat. Transplantation 1965;3:22.
85. Converse JM, Smahel J, Ballantyne DL, et al. Inosculation of vessels of skin graft and host bed: a fortuitous encounter. Br J Plast Surg 1975;28:274.
86. Hynes W. The early circulation in skin grafts with a consideration of methods to encourage their survival. Br J Plast Surg 1954;6:257–63.
87. Hynes W. The skin-dermis graft as an alternative to the direct or tubed flap. Br J Plast Surg 1954;7:97.
88. Rudolph R, Klein L. Healing processes in skin grafts. Surg Gynecol Obstet 1973;136:641654.

89. Smahel J. The healing of skin grafts. Clin Past Surg 1977;4:409–24.

90. Ruffieux P, Hommel L, Saurat J. Long-term assessment of chronic leg ulcer treatment by autologous skin grafts. Dermatology 1997;195:77–80.

91. Plenat F, Vignaud J, Guerret-Stocker S, et al. Host-donor interactions in healing of human split-thickness skin grafts onto nude mice: in situ hybridization, immunohistochemical, and histochemical studies. Transplantation 1992;53:1002–10.

92. Santoni-Rugiu P. An experimental study on the reinnervation of free skin grafts and pedicle flaps. Plast Reconstr Surg 1966;38:98–104.

93. Attinger CE. Use of skin grafting in the foot. J Am Podiatr Med Assoc 1995;85(1):49–56.

94. Branham G, Thomas J. Skin grafts. Otolaryngol Clin North Am 1990;23(5):889–97.

95. Rudolph R. Inhibition of myofibroblasts by skin grafts. Plast Reconstr Surg 1979;63:473480.

96. Davis JS, Kitlowski EA. The immediate contraction of cutaneous grafts and its cause. Arch Surg 1931;23:954.

97. Grabb WC, Smith JW. Basic techniques of plastic surgery. In: Grabb WC, Smith JW, editors. Plastic surgery: a concise guide to clinical practice. Boston: Little, Brown and Company; 1968.

98. Donato M, Novicki DC, Blume PA. Skin grafting techniques for foot and ankle surgeons, clinics in podiatric medicine and surgery, part II. 17(4):2000.

99. Priest RE, Bublitz C. The influence of ascorbic acid and tetrahydropterine on the synthesis of hydroxyproline by cultured cells. Lab Invest 1967;17:371.

100. Evans GR, Robb GL. Cutaneous foot malignancies: outcome and options for reconstruction. Ann Plast Surg 1995;34:396–401.

101. Hutchinson BL. Malignant melanoma in the lower extremity: a comprehensive overview. Clin Podiatr Med Surg 1986;3:533–51.

102. Rowsell AR, Godfrey AM. A fortuitous donor site for full-thickness skin grafts in the correction of syndactyly. Br J Plast Surg 1984;37:31–4.

103. Spence RJ, Wong L. The enhancement of wound healing with human skin allograft. Surg Clin North Am 1997;77:731–42.

104. Stotter A, McLean NR, Fallowfield ME, et al. Reconstruction after excision of soft tissue sarcomas of the limbs and trunk. Br J Surg 1988;75:774–8.

105. Wexler MR, Barlev A, Peled IJ. Plantar split-thickness skin grafts for coverage of superficial pressure ulcers of the foot. J Dermatol Surg Oncol 1983;9:162–4.

106. Weltering EA, Thorpe WP, Reed JK, et al. Split thickness skin grafting of the plantar surface of the foot after wide excision of neoplasms of the skin. Surg Gynecol Obstet 1979;149:229–32.

107. Schroeder SM, Sumpio BE, Blume PA. Poster Presentation, American College of Foot and Ankle Surgeons, 2/04, San Diego California; Double Blind Pilot Study to Evaluate Prewounding Prior to Split Thickness Skin Grafting using Becaplermin Gel, Versus Placebo Gel, and Standard Wound Care with Saline Wet to Dry Dressings.

108. KCI, Inc. P.O. Box 659508, San Antonio (TX) 78265–9508, Protocol VAC 2001–03, A Randomized, Controlled Multicenter Trial Of Vacuum Assisted Closure Therapy With Split Thickness Skin Grafting in the Treatment and Blinded Evaluation of Venous Stasis Ulcers. 10/03.

109. Gilliland EL, Nathwani N, Dore CJ, et al. Bacterial colonisation of leg ulcers and its effect on the success rate of skin grafting. Ann R Coll Surg Engl 1988;70:105–8.

110. Robson MC. Wound infection: a failure of wound healing caused by an imbalance of bacteria. Surg Clin North Am 1997;77:637–50.
111. Deitch EA. Prospective study of the effect of the recipient bed on skin graft survival after thermal injury. J Trauma 1985;25:118–21.
112. Cohen IK, Crossland MC, Garrett A, et al. Topical application of epidermal growth factor onto partial-thickness wounds in human volunteers does not enhance reepithelialization. Plast Reconstr Surg 1995;96:251–4.
113. Fraser GL, Beaulieu JT. Leukopenia secondary to sulfadiazine silver. JAMA 1979;241:1928–9.
114. Van Den Hoogenband HM. Treatment of leg ulcers with split-thickness skin grafts. J Dermatol Surg Oncol 1984;10:605–8.
115. Chu CY, Peng FC, Chiu YF, et al. Nanohybrids of silver particles immobilized on silicate platelet for infected wound healing. PLoS One 2012;7(6): e3836.
116. Smoot EC, Kucan JO, Roth A, et al. In vitro toxicity testing for antibacterials against human keratinocytes. Plast Reconstr Surg 1991;87:917–24.
117. Culliton P, Kwasnik RE, Novicki D, et al. The efficacy of porcine skin grafts for treating non-healing cutaneous ulcers, part 1: clinical studies. J Am Podiatr Med Assoc 1978;68(1):1–11.
118. Marcinko DE, Pentin-Maki R. Wound healing, surgical decompression, and soft tissue coverage in the infected foot. In: Marcinko DE, editor. Infections of the Foot. St Louis (MO): Elsevier - Health Sciences Division; 1998. p. 215–21.
119. Wardrop PJ, Nishikawa H. Lateral cutaneous nerve of the thigh blockade as primary anaesthesia for harvesting skin grafts. Br J Plast Surg 1995;48: 597–600.
120. Sharpe DT, Cardoso E, Baheti V. The immediate mobilisation of patients with lower limb skin grafts: a clinical report. Br J Plast Surg 1983;36:105–8.
121. Kirsner RS, Falanga V. Techniques of split-thickness skin grafting for lower extremity ulcerations. J Dermatol Surg Oncol 1993;19:779–83.
122. Kirsner RS, Mata SM, Falanga V, et al. Split-thickness skin grafting of leg ulcers: the University of Miami Department of Dermatology's Experience (1990–1993). Dermatol Surg 1995;21:701–3.
123. Mahajan R, Mosley JG. Use of a semipermeable polyan-dde dressing over skin grafts to venous leg ulcers. Br J Surg 1995;82:1359–60.
124. Lukash FN. Microvascular free muscle reconstruction of a large plantar defect. Ann Plast Surg 1985;15:252–6.
125. Mahan KT. Plastic surgery and skin grafting. In: McGlamry ED, Banks AS, Downey MS, editors. Comprehensive textbook of foot surgery. 2nd edition. Baltimore (MD): Williams & Wilkins; 1992. p. 1256–96.
126. Carson SN, Overall K, Lee-Jahshan S, et al. Vacuum-assisted closure used for healing chronic wounds and skin grafts in the lower extremities. Ostomy Wound Manage 2004;50(3):52–8.
127. Scherer LA, Shiver S, Chang M, et al. The vacuum assisted closure device: a method of securing skin grafts and improving graft survival. Arch Surg 2002; 137(8):930–4.
128. Schneider AM, Morykwas MJ, Argenta LC. A new and reliable method of securing skin grafts to the difficult recipient bed. Plast Reconstr Surg 1998; 102(4):1195–8.
129. Gupta S. Optimal use of negative pressure wound therapy for skin grafts. Int Wound J 2012;9(1):40–7.

130. Hegelson MD, Potter BK, Evans KN, et al. Bioartificial dermal substitute: a preliminary report on its use for the management of complex combat-related soft tissue wounds. J Orthop Trauma 2007;21(6):394–9.
131. Llanos S, Danilla S, Barraza C, et al. Effectiveness of negative pressure closure in the integration of split thickness skin grafts: a randomized, double-masked, controlled trial. Ann Surg 2006;244(5):700–5.
132. Webster J, Scuffham P, Sherriff KL, et al. Negative pressure wound therapy for skin grafts and surgical wounds healing by primary intention. Cochrane Database Syst Rev 2012;(4):CD009261.
133. Turcic J, Hancevic J, Antoljak T, et al. Effects of ozone on how well split-thickness skin grafts according to Thiersch take in war wounds: results of prospective study. Langenbecks Arch Chir 1995;380:144–8.
134. Egan CA, Gerwels JW. Surgical pearl: use of a sponge bolster instead of a tie-over bolster as a less invasive method of securing full-thickness skin grafts. J Am Acad Dermatol 1998;39:1000–1.
135. Powers KB, Vacek JL, Lee S. Noninvasive approaches to peripheral vascular disease: what's new in evaluation and treatment? Postgrad Med 1999;106:3.
136. Zierler RE, Sumner DS. Physiologic assessment of peripheral arterial occlusive disease. In: Rutherford RB, editor. Vasc Surg. Philadelphia, PA: WB Saunders; 1998. p. 65–117.
137. Horowitz JH, Nichter LS, Kenney JG, et al. Lawnmower injuries in children: lower extremity reconstruction. J Trauma 1985;25:1138–46.
138. Myerson M. Split-thickness skin excision: Its use for immediate wound care in crush injuries of the foot. Foot Ankle 1989;10:54–60.
139. Souther SG. Skin grafts from the sole of the foot: case report and literature review. J Trauma 1980;20:163–5.
140. Wyble EJ, Yakuboff KP, Clark RG, et al. Use of free fasciocutaneous and muscle flaps for reconstruction of the foot. Ann Plast Surg 1990;24:101–8.
141. Golminz D, Bennett RG. Cigarette smoking and flap and full thickness graft necrosis. Arch Dermatol 1982;127:1012.
142. Sanstead H, Shepard G. The effect of zinc deficiency on the tensile strength of healing surgical incisions in the integument of the rat. Proc Soc Exp Biol Med 1968;128:687.

Charcot Neuroarthropathy of the Foot and Ankle

Diagnosis and Management Strategies

Peter A. Blume, DPM[a],*, Bauer Sumpio, MD, PhD[b],
Brian Schmidt, DPM[c], Ryan Donegan, DPM, MS[c]

KEYWORDS

- Charcot osteoarthropathy • Charcot foot • Charcot ankle • Osteomyelitis

KEY POINTS

- Treatment of Charcot osteoarthropathy with and without osteomyelitis is a complex problem requiring a team approach.
- Diagnostically differentiating Charcot osteoarthropathy from osteomyelitis, or concurrent with osteomyelitis requires a multi modal approach.
- Cure of osteomyelitis is ideal when attempting Charcot osteoarthropathy reconstruction.
- Limb salvage of Charcot osteoarthropathy requires an aggressive approach to management.

CHARCOT FOOT AND ANKLE
History of Charcot

Charcot osteoarthropathy was first described more than 140 years ago.[1] Despite the time that has passed since the first publication in 1883, Charcot joint disease of the foot and ankle remains a poorly understood and frequently overlooked complication of diabetes. Recognition, especially in the earliest stage, remains problematic, with many cases being misdiagnosed. J.M. Charcot was the first to describe these arthropathies, associated with tabes dorsalis.[2] His early investigations into the tabetic arthropathies (1868) and his presentation, "Demonstration of Arthropathic Affections of Locomotor Ataxy," at the Seventh International Medical Congress (1881), established the disease as a distinct pathologic entity. Charcot and Féré published the first observations of the tabetic foot in the *Archives de Neurologie* in 1883. It was not until

The authors have no financial sources to disclose.

[a] Orthopedics and Rehabilitation, and Anesthesia, Yale School of Medicine, 20 York Street, New Haven, CT 06510, USA; [b] Section of Vascular Surgery, Department of Surgery, Yale School of Medicine, 20 York Street, New Haven, CT 06510, USA; [c] Section of Podiatric Surgery, Department of Orthopedics and Rehabilitation, Yale New Haven Hospital, 20 York Street, New Haven, CT 06510, USA
* Corresponding author. 508 Blake Street, New Haven, CT 06515.
E-mail address: peter.b@snet.net

Clin Podiatr Med Surg 31 (2014) 151–172
http://dx.doi.org/10.1016/j.cpm.2013.09.007
0891-8422/14/$ – see front matter © 2014 Elsevier Inc. All rights reserved.

podiatric.theclinics.com

1936, however, that W.R. Jordan established the association between neurogenic arthropathy of the foot/ankle and diabetes mellitus. Much of what is known about Charcot today came from initially studying patients with syphilis and leprosy, although diabetes has now become the leading cause of the disorder.

Definition of Charcot Osteoarthropathy

The prevalence of diabetes mellitus is growing at epidemic proportions in the United States and worldwide. The prevalence of diabetes for all age groups worldwide was estimated to be 2.8% in 2000 and will reach 4.4% in 2030.[3] An estimated 7% of the United States population has diabetes, and because of the increased longevity of this population, diabetes-associated complications are expected to increase in prevalence.[4] Foot ulcerations, infections, peripheral arterial disease, and Charcot osteoarthropathy are among the most common diabetic complications, which frequently result in lower limb amputations. The prevalence of neuropathy in patients with and without diabetes mellitus is 77.2% and 11.7%, respectively.[5] Patients with diabetic neuropathy have been found to be older, with poorer glycemic control and higher serum creatinine levels, and reportedly more significant tobacco use than diabetic patients without neuropathy.[5]

Charcot osteoarthropathy is a relatively painless, progressive, and degenerative arthropathy of single or multiple joints caused by underlying neurologic deficits, with peripheral joints most commonly affected. Charcot osteoarthropathy presents as a warm, swollen, erythematous foot and ankle, many times clinically indistinguishable from infection. Current estimates of prevalence range from 0.08% in the general diabetic population to 13% in high-risk diabetic patients.[5] Charcot osteoarthropathy usually occurs 8 to 12 years after the diagnosis of diabetes, during the fifth and sixth decades, with men more frequently affected than women, and a 30% incidence of bilateral involvement.[5]

Etiology of Charcot Osteoarthropathy

All people with Charcot osteoarthropathy have a single common factor, autonomic neuropathy, with diabetes being the most prevalent cause of this condition.[6] The pathogenic mechanism of diabetic neuropathy is a chronic state of hyperglycemia along with microvascular disease, with these 2 processes leading to nerve injury through osmotic changes and ischemia.

Two pathologic theories have gained most acceptance as an explanation of Charcot osteoarthropathy, namely the neurovascular and neurotraumatic. The neurotraumatic theory states that because of unperceived pain sensation, repeated minor trauma occurs in the pedal bones, leading to multiple fractures and collapse of normal pedal architecture. The trauma can result from daily activities, infection, and even recent surgery. In the United Kingdom and Ireland, 36% of patients reported some form of traumatic event, and 12% reported foot surgery during the preceding 6 months of an acute Charcot foot.[7] Chantelau and colleagues,[8] using magnetic resonance imaging (MRI), documented bone trauma in the earliest stages of Charcot foot, providing further evidence to reinforce the role of unperceived trauma. More recently, Chantelau and colleagues[9] found a high threshold for perception of cutaneous pressure pain in Charcot feet, and suggested that these patients fail to perceive inflammatory pain caused by trauma.

The neurovascular theory has become more accepted as the more likely pathologic process. This theory states that destruction of bone occurs secondary to a hypervascular state, which exists secondary to loss of sympathetic function. Blood flow has been proved to be 5 times greater in the neuropathic foot than in the nonneuropathic foot.[10] Autonomic neuropathy results in impaired vascular reflexes with arteriovenous shunting and increased arterial perfusion, which has been demonstrated in both neuropathic foot and acute Charcot foot.[6] It has been shown that people who have had an acute Charcot foot exhibit retention of vasodilatory reflexes, in contrast to diabetic individuals with distal symmetrical neuropathy without Charcot osteoarthropathy.[11] It is believed that increased blood flow causes a leaching out of bone minerals, leading to osteopenia and, ultimately, susceptibility to fracture. In normal skin, arteriovenous (AV) anastomoses are kept shut by vasomotor nerves. When autonomic neuropathy is present a loss of vasomotor nerves occurs, causing AV shunting, which leads to inadequate capillary flow that decreases healing of wounds, increased arteriolar flow that causes bounding pulses, and dysfunction to nerves of sweat glands and sensory endings, causing the epidermis to be more liable to blisters.

Of interest, there may be some pathophysiologic differences between Charcot patients with type 1 and type 2 diabetes. Petrova and colleagues[12] found significantly younger age but significantly longer diabetes duration in Charcot patients with type 1 diabetes in comparison with those with type 2. More impressively, the same group[13] found a generalized reduction of bone mineral density in Charcot patients with type 1 diabetes, but not with type 2 diabetes. At the same time, Charcot patients with type 2 diabetes presented with more severe peripheral neuropathy (impaired temperature and vibration perception) than their type 1 diabetes peers (impaired temperature perception but normal vibration sensation).[13] Thus it would seem that the neurotraumatic theory, with severe loss of protective sensation and mechanical stress from weight bearing in the setting of obesity, might apply more to type 2 than to type 1 diabetes.[13] Conversely, the neurovascular theory, with pronounced bone resorption, might apply more to type 1 than to type 2 diabetes, but further information is needed in this area.[13]

A current theory recently gaining popularity states that uncontrolled local inflammation is the cause of Charcot osteoarthropathy.[6] Christensen and colleagues[10] have provided evidence that local hyperemia in the affected Charcot foot is not accompanied by more severe neuropathic deficits in such patients. The investigators suggested that increased blood flow was attributable to excess local inflammation rather than neuropathy per se.[10] Nowadays a markedly excessive local inflammatory response to trauma is known to be elicited in patients with acute Charcot foot.[14–19] In contrast to the local inflammation, there is no systemic inflammatory response.[20] Increased blood flow in foot bones increased bone resorption with reduced bone mineral density, leading to a predilection for fractures secondary to reduced bone mineral density. This finding has been confirmed in patients with Charcot foot, and increased osteoclastic activity has also been documented.[6]

Normally when a bone is fractured it is associated with pain, leading to splinting of the bone, and the increase in proinflammatory cytokines is usually relatively short lived. In the person who develops an acute Charcot foot, the loss of pain sensation allows for uninterrupted ambulation, with repetitive trauma. It has been suggested that this results in continual production of proinflammatory cytokines, receptor activator of nuclear factor κB ligand (RANKL), nuclear factor-κB (NF-κB), and osteoclasts, which in turn leads to continuing local osteolysis.[11] The continued and excessive release of proinflammatory cytokines, including tumor necrosis factor α and interleukin-1β, leads to increased expression of RANKL. RANKL is responsible for initiating the synthesis of the nuclear transcription factor NF-κB, and this in turn stimulates the maturation of osteoclasts from osteoclast precursor cells. The osteoclastic activity leads to osteoporosis in the affected bones; such increased osteoclastic activity is manifested by an increase in their resorptive capacity in vitro.[21] Osteoclasts generated in vitro in the presence of macrophage colony-stimulating factor and RANKL from patients with active Charcot osteoarthropathy have been shown to be more aggressive, and exhibit an increase in their resorptive activity in comparison with osteoclasts from control subjects.

It is possible that peptides normally secreted from nerve terminals are also important in the underlying pathophysiology. Of these, calcitonin gene–related peptide (CGRP) is a likely candidate because it is known to antagonize the synthesis of RANKL. Hence, any reduction of CGRP through nerve damage will result in an increase in RANKL expression. It is of particular interest that CGRP has been reported to be necessary for the maintenance of the normal integrity of joint capsules, and it follows that any reduction in CGRP release by nerve terminals could facilitate joint dislocation. It is intriguing that healthy neurons secrete the beneficial CGRP, which reduces the synthesis of RANKL and contributes to the maintenance of joint integrity.[15,16] It follows that any reduction of CGRP will be detrimental because it will, indirectly, increase the action of RANKL, aggravating the disease process.[15,16] The role of CGRP is particularly relevant in cases of neuropathy, whereby its secretion has been documented to be reduced.[15,16] Hence, it is now deemed most likely that neuropathy adopts a contributory role in the inflammation-induced osteolysis through reduced secretion of CGRP from affected neurons. Young and colleagues[22] have reported more severe neuropathy in Charcot patients than in their neuropathic peers without Charcot foot.

Apart from the presence of neuropathy and possible osteopenia, other contributory factors include the effects of advanced glycosylation end products, reactive oxygen species, and oxidized lipids, all of which may enhance the expression of RANKL in diabetes. The effect of local inflammation on this pathway would similarly compound the expression of RANKL. Other cases may be triggered by different causes of local inflammation, including previous ulceration, infection, or recent foot surgery. Some other factors have been also implicated in the pathophysiology of the Charcot foot,[14] the most important of which include increased nonenzymatic collagen glycation and elevated plantar pressures. Nonenzymatic collagen glycation may lead to shortening of the Achilles tendon, which in turn will increase forefoot pressures, predisposing to trauma and bone destruction.[23] Elevated plantar pressures have been found in patients with acute Charcot foot, in contrast to their counterparts without Charcot.[24]

DIAGNOSING CHARCOT OSTEOARTHROPATHY
Clinical Diagnosis

Charcot foot is a diagnosis by clinical examination; imaging should be used to stage and supplement the evaluation of progression. In practical clinical application, the Charcot foot can be classified into the acute and chronic stage.[25–29] In the acute stage the foot is markedly red, warm, and swollen. This abnormality usually affects the midfoot. Pain is not a prominent feature, and patients may report no pain or only some discomfort, which is usually much less in comparison with patients without neuropathy and a similar degree of local inflammation.[25–27] The average initial temperature difference between the affected site and a similar site of the contralateral foot is reported as 3.04 C.[25–28,30,31] If the condition is correctly diagnosed and the patient is appropriately immobilized, the local inflammation will subside, and further bony destruction including progressive loss of mineral density can be minimized or avoided.[27,32] By contrast, sustained mechanical stress perpetuates the disease process and may lead to ligament strain, fracture-dislocations of forefoot bones, midfoot collapse, and severe foot deformity and/or joint instability.[25–27,32,33] Charcot osteoarthropathy has increased bone turnover. Some studies have found the carboxyl-terminal telopeptide region of type 1 collagen[11] and bone-specific alkaline phosphatase to be useful markers of bone turnover in patients with Charcot osteoarthropathy.[31] These markers are often used as indicators of disease activity and to measure the response to therapeutic agents. However, because they are not specific for Charcot osteoarthropathy, they are not of particular use for its diagnosis.[11]

Imaging Modalities for Diagnosis

In acute Charcot, which Shibata coined stage 0,[34] only MRI can reveal inflammation of the bone (subchondral bone marrow edema with or without microfracture) and of adjacent soft tissue. In the earliest stage, no radiographic changes are observed. The utility of this knowledge for an early diagnosis at this stage is critical in preventing long-term sequelae. MRI was also used to confirm the recovery from the acute phase through the disappearance of the bone edema, and to verify the absence of any bone fracture.[31] MRI shows typical signs in stage 0 and offers the highest diagnostic accuracy; in fact it is recommended for diagnosing Charcot osteoarthropathy, especially in the early stages.[13,35,36] Zampa and colleagues[37] measured the uptake of contrast medium (gadolinium) on dynamic MRI in 40 patients with acute Charcot osteoarthropathy, and found this to be a reliable means of monitoring the treatment outcome in the acute stage. In a study by Ruotolo and colleagues,[38] all patients showed increased uptake of ^{18}F-fluorodeoxyglucose (FDG) in the Charcot foot. At baseline, the maximum standardized uptake value (SUV_{max}) was significantly higher than the corresponding area in the contralateral foot. Images from positron emission tomography/computed tomography (PET/CT) scans may also be useful for diagnosing stage 0 Charcot osteoarthropathy by highlighting the presence of an area, or several areas, with increased metabolism. In addition, the possibility to quantify this metabolism by calculating SUV_{max} offers the unique opportunity to have an objective evaluation of the intensity of the inflammatory process and the possibility to follow up its evolution. The 2011 American Diabetes Association Consensus on Charcot osteoarthropathy underlines that the duration and aggressiveness of offloading are guided by clinical assessment of the inflammatory process, and that healing of Charcot osteoarthropathy is based on the disappearance of edema, erythema, and a decrease in changes of skin temperature. The study by Ruotolo and colleagues[38] shows that clinical criteria can be misleading, and that such criteria alone are insufficient to establish the time at which the inflammatory process is truly over. By contrast, PET/CT is useful in establishing when the acute active stage has settled and when weight bearing may be allowed once again. Ruotolo and colleagues[38] found signs of inflammation on PET/CT for an average duration of 15 months. From this study, PET/CT scanning in conjunction with MRI may be useful to help diagnose acute Charcot osteoarthropathy.

Diagnosing Charcot osteoarthropathy is most complicated when there is concern for osteomyelitis, which occurs in 20% of diabetic patients.[39] The most difficult differentiation is Charcot osteoarthropathy, osteomyelitis, and Charcot osteoarthropathy with concurrent osteomyelitis. In Charcot osteoarthropathy, MRI shows low signal intensity in subchondral bone on both T1-weighted and T2-weighted images; this appearance correlates with sclerosis on radiographs. By contrast, in osteomyelitis there is low signal intensity on T1-weighted images and high signal intensity on T2-weighted images.[40] On MRI, a Charcot foot will show localized juxta-articular edema, whereas in osteomyelitis the edema is more on one side of the joint and is not confined to the juxta-articular area.[40] Clinically, osteomyelitis affects a single bone in the forefoot or hindfoot, whereas Charcot osteoarthropathy affects many bones, commonly in the midfoot.[41] PET has been recently advocated for differentiating between early-stage Charcot osteoarthropathy and osteomyelitis.[42–44] PET has a distinct advantage over MRI in patients with metal implants. Addition of FDG further adds to the diagnostic capability of PET.[11] Zhuang and colleagues[45] found FDG PET to be 100% sensitive and 87.5% specific for excluding chronic osteomyelitis. Basu and colleagues[43] found FDG PET to have a high negative predictive value in ruling out infection in diabetic patients with foot ulcers. The overall accuracy of MRI for the diagnosis of osteomyelitis is 89%.[41] MRI has gained considerable favor because it allows simultaneous evaluation of soft tissue and osseous structures for infective processes, as well as defining the anatomic location of infected tissue with good accuracy and localization.[46] One study investigated single-photon emission CT in combination with CT, coupled with bedside percutaneous bone biopsy when a positive scan was obtained. The sensitivity and specificity of this combined method were 88.0% and 93.6%, respectively, and the positive and negative predictive values were 91.7% and 90.7%, respectively.[46]

Laboratory Diagnosis

A meta-analysis concluded that the gold standard for the diagnosis of osteomyelitis was bone biopsy. Surgical percutaneous bone biopsy after a 14-day antibiotic-free period represents the gold standard of care for diabetic foot osteomyelitis, but may be difficult to implement in many institutions. Culture of bone specimens was positive in 96% of patients. The identification of a causative organism by culture both confirms osteomyelitis and allows tailoring of antimicrobial therapy; however, cultures from samples obtained during surgery or by imaging guidance are often negative. Several studies suggest that 40% to 60% of histologically proven cases of osteomyelitis at surgery or biopsy are negative at culture.[47] Weiner and colleagues[48] conducted a study to test the claim that there is no difference between histology and microbiology with regard to making the diagnosis of pedal osteomyelitis in diabetic patients. Their results showed that a positive microbiological and negative histologic result was just as likely as a negative microbiological and positive histologic result.

TREATMENT PROTOCOL

Historically, early offloading of the affected foot has been the essential treatment measure for acute Charcot osteoarthropathy. The aim of treatment is to immobilize the affected foot until inflammation has subsided and the fractures have healed. A total contact cast (TCC) for offloading the affected foot during the acute phase is currently the most favored conservative therapy. Pinzur and colleagues[49] recommended weight bearing with a TCC for the initial 6 to 8 weeks, with biweekly change of cast, for acute Charcot osteoarthropathy. Based on a retrospective study, de Souza[50] also recommended a weight-bearing TCC for the acute stage of Charcot osteoarthropathy. The recommended duration of immobilization in accordance with most of the studies on Charcot osteoarthropathy is 4 to 6 months. However, Clohisy and Thompson[51] highlighted the risk of fracture resulting from increased stress on the contralateral weight-bearing limb.

The location of the arthropathy also determines for how long the TCC is indicated. Sinacore[52] stated that forefoot arthropathy heals faster than that of the ankle, midfoot, and hindfoot when TCC is used. It is recommended that immobilization be maintained until a temperature difference of less than 2°C between the affected and nonaffected foot.[53] Because the bones are fragile and joints are usually stiff after the initial immobilization, gradual restoration to full weight bearing is advised, starting with partial weight bearing. Vigorous mobilization can cause relapse of the disease process and is therefore to be avoided.[11]

Adjunctive Therapy

Bisphosphonates have shown some promise in the acute stage of Charcot osteoarthropathy, although the evidence is inconclusive. One study found intranasal calcitonin to be effective in arresting excessive bone turnover in patients with acute Charcot osteoarthropathy.[54] Further larger clinical trials are required to establish the benefits of the pharmacologic agents recommended for Charcot osteoarthropathy.[55–58]

Recurrence After Treatment

In the past, recurrence of Charcot osteoarthropathy was believed to occur only infrequently. By contrast, the few recent studies touching on recurrence of Charcot osteoarthropathy report recurrence rates of from 12% to 33%.[53,59,60] Fabrin and colleagues[60] reported recurrence rates exceeding 15% when treated conservatively. In one series, the recurrence rate of Charcot osteoarthropathy in the ipsilateral foot was 7.1%[6] Recurrence of osteoarthropathic activity was seen in 23% of patients. The mean interval between the end of initial immobilization and orthopedic footwear or orthotic treatment and onset of recurrent Charcot osteoarthropathy was 27 months. Predictors of recurrence were noncompliance and obesity.[31] Sensitivity of the factor "noncompliance" in predicting recurrence was 69% and specificity 90%. The second significant factor to predict the chance of recurrence, with sensitivity of 54% and specificity of 85%, was obesity. Patients with a body mass index of greater than 30 kg/m^2 had an odds ratio of 6.4 to experience recurrence of active Charcot osteoarthropathy. Patients with recurrence were immobilized for a shorter period of time and had a more advanced stage of Charcot osteoarthropathy at the time of first diagnosis. Localization according to Sanders and Frykberg,[61] and stage of disease according to Eichenholtz,[62] were documented. The most frequent localization of osteoarthropathic activity and destruction was the Chopart and Lisfranc joint. The localization of the second attack of Charcot osteoarthropathy was seen in the same area of the foot in 7 of 13 feet, in the same area and an adjacent level according to Sanders' localization in 4 of 13 feet, and in a different region of the foot in 2 of 13 feet. Twelve of 13 feet (92%) that showed signs of recurrence at follow-up had an advanced stage of Charcot osteoarthropathy (Eichenholtz stage >0) at the time of first diagnosis, versus 79% in the group without recurrence.[31] To avoid recurrence of Charcot osteoarthropathy, it is recommend that imaging methods such as MRI or bone scintigraphy be used before discontinuation of immobilization.[53,63,64] This high recurrence rate supports surgical intervention for Charcot osteoarthropathy.

Goals of Surgical Treatment

Traditionally, surgery has been reserved for after quiescence and consolidation, and only if gross deformity is present. Conservative treatment in many instances does not address the pathology sufficiently enough, leading to further complications and inadequate treatment. Surgery is usually reserved for patients in whom conservative treatment has failed, or for treating complications such as deformity, joint instability, infection, and recurrent ulceration associated with bony deformities or contractures; chronic pain; and acute displaced fractures in neuropathic patients with adequate circulation (**Figs. 1** and **2**). Gross instability at the tarsometatarsal articulation will lead to

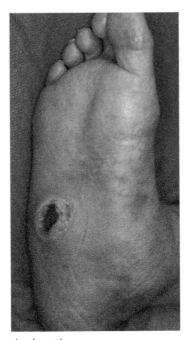

Fig. 1. Deformity with chronic ulceration.

the characteristic symptomatic medial and plantar bony prominences, which can cause ulceration and infection, often resulting in amputation of the limb. Originally the only option was amputation after conservative treatment, such as bracing and appropriate shoe wear, had failed. The aim of surgery is, therefore, to achieve a plantigrade foot with normal distribution of plantar pressure. Saltzman and colleagues[65] reported that nonoperative treatment is associated with an approximately 2.7% annual rate of amputation, a 23% risk of requiring bracing for more than 18 months, and a 49% risk of recurrent ulceration. However, amputation, in addition to the effect of the loss of limb, puts the patient at additional risk of amputation of the contralateral limb. In addition, because of the energy costs, patients often adapt their lifestyle by becoming less active, resulting in reduced physical conditioning of the muscles of the remaining lower extremity.[66–68] Pinzur[69] demonstrated that energy consumption with a unilateral amputation is directly proportional to the number of functional joints remaining and inversely proportional to the length of the remaining limb. Furthermore, Waters and colleagues[68] demonstrated that energy consumption increases 10% to

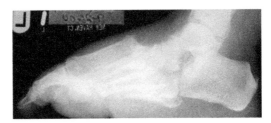

Fig. 2. Osseous deformity.

40% with a unilateral below-the-knee amputation, and 50% to 70% with a unilateral above-the-knee amputation. For this reason, limb salvage is important.

The aim of surgery is to stabilize and align the foot/ankle and make it amenable to wearing appropriate braces or footwear (**Figs. 3** and **4**). The options for surgical treatment range from exostectomy and soft-tissue balancing to internal fixation, intramedullary beaming, external fixation, and gradual correction with a spatial frame. Surgical treatment of Charcot is riddled with potential complications, such as large spatial defects from either joint destruction or resection of osteomyelitis, localized osteoporotic bone, hardware failure, long-standing deformities, chronic soft-tissue contractures, peripheral scarring of the neurovascular bundle, poor wound healing, nonunion, and recurrence of deformity. The surgeon has a plethora of surgical options to address these complications. Large spatial defects can be successfully reconstructed with bone grafting. Localized osteoporotic bone can be treated with external fixation. Long-standing deformities, chronic soft-tissue contractures, and peripheral scarring of the neurovascular bundle can be gradually corrected with spatial frames. Ostectomy alone does not address the biomechanical instability, and thus does not provide long-term benefit. Today, with the advancements in technique and fixation, surgical reconstruction is possible. The primary goal of surgical treatment is to create a functional plantigrade foot that allows the patient to return to functional activity, prevent additional breakdown, and decrease the medical costs.

Neuropathic deformities impair joint mobility in the foot and ankle, often leading to abnormal stresses and impact forces. Sinacore and colleagues[70] determined differences in radiographic measures of hindfoot alignment and the motion of ankle and subtalar joints in participants with and without neuropathic midfoot deformities. The investigators found that an increasing talar declination angle and a decreasing calcaneal inclination angle is associated with decreases in ankle-joint plantarflexion in individuals with neuropathic midfoot deformity because of Charcot neuroarthropathy that

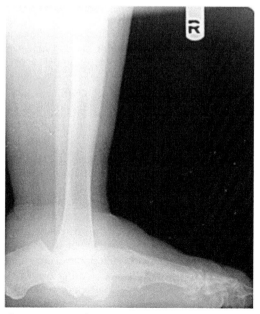

Fig. 3. Deformity before reconstruction.

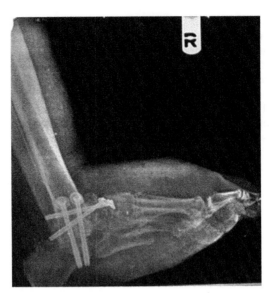

Fig. 4. Deformity reconstructed to prevent recurrent wounds.

may contribute to excessive stresses and, ultimately, plantar ulceration of the midfoot. Moreover, subjects with talonavicular and calcaneocuboid dislocations experienced the most severe restrictions in ankle-joint plantarflexion and inversion motions of the subtalar joint.[71] The tarsometatarsal articulation is the most common location for the development of neuropathic arthropathy, with 60% to 70% of cases at this location,[72] followed by the hindfoot, ankle joint, and forefoot. Destruction of the Lisfranc joint complex causes rocker bottom deformity, leading to plantar ulceration, which, especially in the course of diabetes, often results in infection and significant morbidity. Minimizing soft-tissue damage during surgery is essential, because incomplete or slow healing is generally known to be associated with neuropathy, vasculopathy, dermopathy, and difficulty avoiding weight-bearing activities, all of which are known to affect this patient population. Rigid osteosynthesis is also important, owing to the high likelihood of uncontrolled postoperative weight bearing, which can lead to failure of the implants and reconstruction.[73] Therefore, the goal of reconstruction should be to achieve the radiographic measurements reported in the aforementioned studies, and to prevent ulceration.

Adjunctive Surgical Procedures

According to the Brodsky classification, Type 1 (midfoot) involvement commonly leads to formation of these problematic bony prominences.[74] In patients with deformity, exostectomy is a viable option provided the midfoot deformity is stable; otherwise, there is a risk of worsening the deformity.[74–76] Garapati and Weinfeld[75] recommended an operative approach via separate incisions on the non–weight-bearing surface of the foot. Furthermore, they advocated going through the ulcer for centrally located prominences, and primary closure of any small and superficial ulcers during exostectomy. Many investigators have recommended lengthening the Achilles tendon in cases of recurrent ulceration and equinus deformity, which decreases stress across midfoot joints by increasing the calcaneal inclination angle.[77,78] Mueller and colleagues[79] performed a randomized controlled trial to compare the recurrence rate of ulceration in patients with neuropathic plantar ulcers treated with Achilles-tendon lengthening plus total contact casting, and a TCC alone. At 7 months' follow-up a 15% ulcer recurrence in the group with Achilles-tendon lengthening plus total contact casting was reported, compared with 59% in the group with total contact casting alone. In Charcot feet with ulcers, the procedure can be staged with initial debridement and an external fixator, followed by an internal fixator and bone grafting.

Autografts required for arthrodeses can be harvested from iliac crest, tibia, or fibula. Hollawell[80] recommended the use of the allogenic cellular bone matrix Osteocel Plus as an autograft alternative in cases of high-risk ankle and foot arthrodesis. At the end of 6 months he reported 100% radiologic fusion. However, only 3 patients with Charcot osteoarthropathy were included in the study. Adequate autologous bone grafting is used after preparing the joint surfaces.

Fixation for Surgical Reconstruction

The choice of implant for arthrodesis depends on the surgeon's preference, as none has been proved to be superior to others. Screws, plates, intramedullary devices, and external fixators have all been used for arthrodesis. In a retrospective study, Grant and colleagues[81] highlighted the stability of a construct using large stainless-steel intramedullary screws as beams for lateral and medial columns along with arthrodesis of the subtalar joint for reconstruction of Charcot feet. Sammarco[82] used the term "superconstructs" for a combination of plantar plating, locking-plate technology, and axial screw fixation during reconstruction of midfoot deformities in Charcot feet. These superconstructs entail extending the fusion beyond the affected zone by inclusion of nonaffected joints, reduction of deformity without causing excessive soft-tissue tension by shortening the extremity, using the strongest devices that can be tolerated by the soft-tissue envelope, and applying the device in the optimal position to increase mechanical function. External fixators have been advocated by many investigators,[83–85] with the main advantage being the ability to monitor soft-tissue healing and avoidance of more invasive surgery in patients with infection. However, their main drawback is pin-tract infection. External fixation is known to be associated with a substantial risk of pin-site infection and patient inconvenience owing to the prominence of the frame. The key advantage of this method is that a long incision and wide exposure are not required for fixation.

Lamm and colleagues[86] recommended a staged minimally invasive technique whereby initially an external fixator is applied for gradual distraction followed by arthrodesis using percutaneous internal fixation. Altindas and colleagues[87] reported a 2-stage Boyd operation technique for late-stage Charcot feet. Most of the patients in their study had hindfoot involvement. The first stage includes talectomy, joint surface preparation (for calcaneotibial arthrodesis), and fixation of the calcaneum to the tibia with Kirschner wires after fashioning the joint surface and pushing the calcaneum forward. Second-stage closure of the flaps is performed 2 to 3 weeks later. The investigators reported no complications, with a mean follow-up of 2.1 years.

Simon and colleagues[88] performed arthrodesis of the tarsal-metatarsal region in 14 patients with Eichenholtz stage 1 Charcot feet, and reported 100% success rate without any postoperative complications.

Garchar and colleagues[71] have shown good clinical outcomes from plantar plating the medial midfoot, first metatarsal, medial cuneiform, and navicular, as well as for Lisfranc dislocation in Charcot neuropathy. These investigators achieved a 96% union rate, with an average time to ambulation of 11.68 weeks. Wiewiorski and colleagues[89] showed successful restoration of alignment of the medial column (medial metatarsocuneiform, medial naviculocuneiform, and talonavicular joints) with intramedullary placement of a 6.5-mm diameter solid bolt, with a mean American Orthopaedic Foot and Ankle Society midfoot score of 67 at final follow-up. All patients were able to walk at least 1 block at the final follow-up visit, and no cases of recurrent or residual ulceration developed. At a mean follow-up duration of 27 months no bolt breakage had occurred, and the midfoot alignment was maintained in all but 1 patient, in whom postoperative infection caused massive osteolysis and failure. None of the patients experienced postoperative ulceration or amputation during the observation period. Sammarco and colleagues[82] used 6.5-mm cannulated screws and reported breakage of the screws in 8 (36.4%) of 22 cases. Research has shown that a plate applied to the plantar (tension) aspect of the medial midfoot provides a stronger, sturdier construct than midfoot fusion with screw fixation.[90] Marks and colleagues[90] demonstrated the biomechanical superiority of plantar plates for midfoot stabilization in a cadaver study, in comparison with solid bolt fixation. However, placement of a plate usually requires extensive dissection and exposure, resulting in accompanying soft-tissue damage. Sammarco[82] has shown impressive clinical results using intramedullary screws; however, screws have a substantial risk of breaking, which Sammarco reported in 36.4% of cases. Drawback of the fusion bolt is the predilection for axial migration, which Wieworski and colleagues[89] observed in 37.5% of patients. In 2 of those patients, the midfoot bolt penetrated into the ankle joint and necessitated subsequent implant removal. Of note, bolt migration occurred only in cases where the intramedullary bolt was used to stabilize the medial column when joint surface resection with the goal of arthrodesis was not performed. Studies have also revealed that a plantar plate allows significantly less initial displacement and maintains stabilization at a much greater load.[90]

Pope and colleagues[73] specifically compared plantar planting with intramedullary screws for midfoot fusion. There was no failure of hardware, and no notable differences between the 2 fixation techniques with respect to stiffness or loads to failure. There was a trend toward a stiffer first tarsometatarsal joint construct using the plantar-plating method. Furthermore, the intramedullary screw construct failed at the first tarsometatarsal joint in 5 of 7 placements, whereas none of the plantar-plating constructs failed at the first tarsometatarsal joint.

Stability of the medial column has been emphasized by multiple investigators. Pinzur and Sostak[91] reported their results on operative stabilization of midfoot Charcot deformities. Their operative indication was a foot that was not plantigrade, based on the lateral talar–first metatarsal angle. The Schon classification assigns a beta stage if 1 of 4 criteria is met, 2 of them being that the lateral talar–first metatarsal angle is 30° or more or the anteroposterior talar–first metatarsal angle is 35° or more.[92] Both of these measurements highlight the importance of medial-column stability.[92] Many different approaches to surgical treatment and reconstruction have shown that medial-column stability is critical.

Charcot Osteoarthropathy with Osteomyelitis

When formulating a treatment algorithm for Charcot osteoarthropathy, it is imperative to address all factors that may have an effect on outcome. The process of reconstruction of Charcot osteoarthropathy in the presence of an open wound requires resection of the wound with elimination of osteomyelitis with antibiotic therapy (intravenous, oral, implantation of bone cement/antibiotic-loaded beads/bone-void filler with antibiotics), and exchange of bone cement or replacement of deficit with bone graft or primary arthrodesis with external fixation. Typically noted in patients with an open wound, negative pressure wound therapy with skin grafting may be necessary. On treating Charcot osteoarthropathy with concurrent osteomyelitis, the primary goal is to achieve as close as possible to full eradication of osteomyelitis before final reconstruction takes place. There are many considerations that affect treatment choices for osteomyelitis, such as bone penetration, method of administration of antibiotics, and duration of treatment, which depends on cleanliness of borders and continuous monitoring of culture-positive and culture-negative wounds. The standard recommendation for treating chronic osteomyelitis is 6 weeks of parenteral antibiotic therapy. However, oral antibiotics that achieve adequate levels in bone have now become available. Oral and parenteral therapies achieve similar cure rates; however, oral therapy avoids risks associated with intravenous catheters and is generally less expensive, making it a reasonable choice for osteomyelitis caused by susceptible organisms.[93] Jeffcoate and Lipsky[94] highlighted that antibiotics alone may apparently eliminate bone infection in many cases. There is also evidence for the effectiveness of local antibiotics in treating osteomyelitis. The use of antimicrobial-loaded bone cement allows for high local doses while avoiding systemic toxicity. The primary benefit achieved with local antibiotic delivery vehicles is the ability to obtain very high levels of local antibiotics without increasing systemic toxicity.[95–99] Regardless of the antibiotic loading dose, the teicoplanin-loaded cements showed better elution efficacy and provided longer inhibitory periods against methicillin-susceptible *Staphylococcus aureus*, methicillin-resistant *S aureus*, and vancomycin-intermediate *S aureus* than did cements loaded with the same dose of vancomycin or daptomycin. For treatment of *S aureus* infection, teicoplanin was superior in terms of antibacterial effects.[100]

Deformity Correction Algorithm

For maintaining deformity correction achieved in reconstruction, Steinmann pins are often used for stabilization with compression from an Ilizarov external fixation for midfoot, hindfoot, and ankle, the goal being complete fusion, although pseudarthrosis can create a stable lower extremity allowing for ambulation and a reduced risk of ulceration/reulceration. A severe diabetic foot infection carries a 25% risk of major amputation.[101] The overall strategy for surgically managing a severe diabetic foot infection is infection control through aggressive and extensive surgical debridement, a comprehensive vascular assessment with possible vascular surgery and/or endovascular intervention, and soft-tissue and skeletal reconstruction after the infection is eradicated, to obtain wound closure and limb salvage[83,102–106] (**Fig. 5**). The largest study

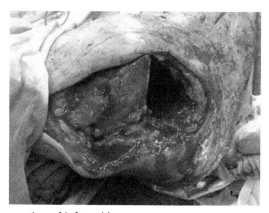

Fig. 5. Aggressive resection of infected bone.

to date involved 73 cases of lower extremity Charcot osteoarthropathy with osteomyelitis, conducted by Pinzur and colleagues,[107] who used a single-stage procedure for treatment. The first step of the surgery involved radical resection of the clinically infected bone. Tissue cultures from the resected bone were used to guide parenteral antibiotic therapy. Sufficient bone was then removed to allow correction of the deformity to a plantigrade position. Large smooth percutaneous pins were used for provisional fixation. Maintenance of the surgically obtained correction was achieved with a 3-level preconstructed static circular external fixator. When the disease process involved the ankle joint, correction was maintained with a similar circular construct, with compression being applied across the ankle joint. Wounds were loosely reapproximated when possible, and managed with adjuvant dressings and wound care when they could not be closed. All patients were treated with culture-specific parenteral antibiotic therapy that was administered and monitored by an infectious disease comanagement consultation service. Both the choice and duration of antibiotic therapy was made by the infectious disease consultant. The circular external fixator was maintained for a period of 8 weeks in patients with deformity in the foot, and a minimum 12 weeks when the ankle was involved. Following removal of the external fixator, patients were managed in a weight-bearing TCC for 4 to 6 weeks, followed by a commercially available diabetic fracture boot. Patients were transitioned to therapeutic footwear consisting of commercially available depth-inlay shoes and custom accommodative foot orthoses. Using this protocol, the investigators were able to achieve 95.7% limb salvage, with ambulation in commercially available therapeutic footwear. (**Figs. 6–8**)

PATIENTS WITH CHARCOT OSTEOARTHROPATHY ARE COMPLEX PATIENTS

Diabetic patients with Charcot osteoarthropathy are complex patients, with many comorbidities other than osteomyelitis. The introduction of the hospitalist comanagement model represents an opportunity to improve care. Pinzur and colleagues[108] conducted a study to investigate the outcomes of diabetic patients undergoing treatment of osteomyelitis and Charcot osteoarthropathy reconstruction after being enrolled in an academic medical center hospitalist–orthopedic surgery comanagement

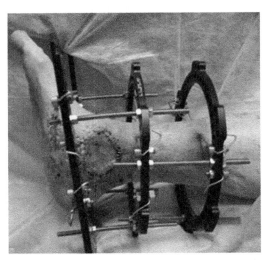

Fig. 6. External fixation with skin graft to maintain surgical construction.

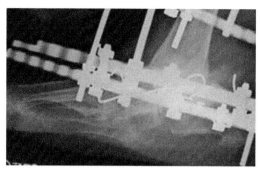

Fig. 7. External fixation maintaining osseous alignment.

patient-care program. While the overall observed-to-expected cost of care remained virtually unchanged, the positive impact of the study model revealed an increased positive effect on the patients more severely affected by severity of illness and risk of mortality. The results of this study suggest that a proactive, cooperative, comanagement model for the perioperative management of high-risk patients undergoing complex surgery can improve the quality and efficiency metrics associated with the delivery of service to patients. Healing of Charcot osteoarthropathy depends on hemoglobin A1c, creatinine, overall comorbidities, underlying systemic arthropathies such as rheumatoid and lupus, chronic prednisone use, end-stage renal disease on hemodialysis, and, for a small percentage of elderly patients, distal revascularization, which is why medical comanagement is crucial for successful outcomes.

Ultimately, there has as yet been no agreement on protocol for treating Charcot osteoarthropathy of the lower extremity with or without osteomyelitis. The most current literature on treatment highlights the lack of consensus, although it does show some commonality among approaches.

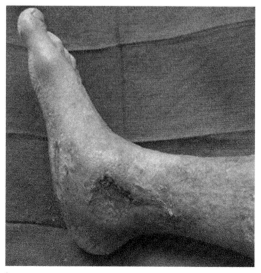

Fig. 8. Salvaged limb.

SUMMARY

The treatment of Charcot osteoarthropathy is an extremely involved and long-term process, many times involving multiple surgeries, antibiotics, extended periods of non–weight bearing and immobilization, and external fixation. It is a huge undertaking, and probably one of the most involved and taxing a patient can undergo both physically and mentally, all without any guarantee of correction or prevention of recurrence. Many patients ultimately need major amputations.

Lower extremity amputation in patients with diabetes is associated with premature mortality and impaired ambulatory status. Despite advances in limb-salvage techniques, certain patients will require major amputation. Significant improvement after transtibial amputation occurred in the SF-36 Physical Component Summary score and the Foot and Ankle Measure Activity of Daily Living. In a select group of Charcot osteoarthropathy patients, transtibial amputation resulted in improvement in self-reported outcomes. Although major lower extremity amputation is a devastating complication in patients with diabetes, there is some low-level evidence that major amputation may be a more practical solution.[109]

The negative impact on health-related quality of life in patients with Charcot osteoarthropathy has prompted operative correction of the acquired deformity. Comparative-effects financial models are being introduced to provide valuable information to assist in clinical decision making. In a recent study by Gil and colleagues,[110] patients with Charcot osteoarthropathy underwent operative correction with the use of circular external fixation. A control group was created from 17 diabetic patients who successfully underwent transtibial amputation and prosthetic fitting during the same period. The cost of care during the 12 months following surgery was derived from inpatient hospitalization, placement in a rehabilitation unit or skilled nursing facility, home health care including parenteral antibiotic therapy, physical therapy, and purchase of prosthetic devices or footwear. Fifty-three of the patients with limb salvage (69.7%) did not require inpatient rehabilitation. Their average cost of care was US$56,712. Fourteen of the patients with amputation (82.4%) required inpatient rehabilitation, at an average cost of $49,251.[110]

Questions that need to be addressed include length of treatment, the impact of long-term immobilization, and whether reconstruction of Charcot osteoarthropathy with osteomyelitis is a better treatment than primary amputation. Perhaps the first study that needs to be performed should pertain to functional scores comparing below-knee amputation with reconstruction, to determine which undertaking is more beneficial for the patient.

This article presents a review of current literature discussing the etiology, pathophysiology, diagnosis and imaging, and conservative and surgical treatment of Charcot osteoarthropathy, as well as the treatment of Charcot osteoarthropathy with concurrent osteomyelitis.

REFERENCES

1. Chisholm KA, Gilchrist JM. The Charcot joint: a modern neurologic perspective. J Clin Neuromuscul Dis 2011;13:1–13.
2. Sanders LJ. The Charcot foot: historical perspective 1827-2003. Diabetes Metab Res Rev 2004;20(Suppl 1):S4–8.
3. Wild S, Roglic G, Green A, et al. Global prevalence of diabetes: estimates for the year 2000 and projections for 2030. Diabetes Care 2004;27: 1047–53.

4. Frykberg RG, Zgonis T, Armstrong DG, et al. Diabetic foot disorders. A clinical practice guideline. J Foot Ankle Surg 2006;45:S1–66.
5. Suder NC, Wukich DK. Prevalence of diabetic neuropathy in patients undergoing foot and ankle surgery. Foot Ankle Spec 2012;5:97–101.
6. Papanas N, Maltezos E. Etiology, pathophysiology and classifications of the diabetic Charcot foot. Diabet Foot Ankle 2013;4:208–72.
7. Game FL, Catlow R, Jones GR, et al. Audit of acute Charcot's disease in the UK: the CDUK study. Diabetologia 2012;55:32–5.
8. Chantelau E, Richter A, Schmidt-Grigoriadis P, et al. The diabetic Charcot foot: MRI discloses bone stress injury as trigger mechanism of neuroarthropathy. Exp Clin Endocrinol Diabetes 2006;114:118–23.
9. Chantelau E, Wienemann T, Richter A. Pressure pain thresholds at the diabetic Charcot-foot: an exploratory study. J Musculoskelet Neuronal Interact 2012;12: 95–101.
10. Christensen TM, Simonsen L, Holstein PE, et al. Sympathetic neuropathy in diabetes mellitus patients does not elicit Charcot osteoarthropathy. J Diabetes Complications 2011;25:320–4.
11. Madan SS, Pai DR. Charcot neuroarthropathy of the foot and ankle. Orthop Surg 2013;5:86–93.
12. Petrova NL, Foster AV, Edmonds ME. Difference in presentation of Charcot osteoarthropathy in type 1 compared with type 2 diabetes. Diabetes Care 2004;27:1235–6.
13. Petrova NL, Foster AV, Edmonds ME. Calcaneal bone mineral density in patients with Charcot neuropathic osteoarthropathy: differences between Type 1 and Type 2 diabetes. Diabet Med 2005;22:756–61.
14. Gouveri E, Papanas N. Charcot osteoarthropathy in diabetes: a brief review with an emphasis on clinical practice. World J Diabetes 2011;2:59–65.
15. Jeffcoate WJ. Review Charcot neuro-osteoarthropathy. Diabetes Metab Res Rev 2008;24:S62–5.
16. Rogers LC, Frykberg RG, Armstrong DG, et al. The Charcot foot in diabetes. Diabetes Care 2011;34:2123–9.
17. Jeffcoate WJ, Game F, Cavanagh PR. The role of proinflammatory cytokines in the cause of neuropathic osteoarthropathy (acute Charcot foot) in diabetes. Lancet 2005;366:2058–61.
18. Jeffcoate W. The causes of the Charcot syndrome. Clin Podiatr Med Surg 2008; 25:29–42.
19. Jeffcoate WJ. Theories concerning the pathogenesis of the acute Charcot foot suggest future therapy. Curr Diab Rep 2005;5:430–5.
20. Petrova NL, Moniz C, Elias DA, et al. Is there a systemic inflammatory response in the acute Charcot foot? Diabetes Care 2007;30:997–8.
21. Mabilleau G, Petrova NL, Edmonds ME, et al. Increased osteoclastic activity in acute Charcot's osteoarthropathy: the role of receptor activator of nuclear factor-kappaB ligand. Diabetologia 2008;51:1035–40.
22. Young MJ, Marshall A, Adams JE, et al. Osteopenia, neurological dysfunction, and the development of Charcot neuroarthropathy. Diabetes Care 1995;18: 34–8.
23. Grant WP, Sullivan R, Sonenshine DE, et al. Electron microscopic investigation of the effects of diabetes mellitus on the Achilles tendon. J Foot Ankle Surg 1997; 36:272–8.
24. Armstrong DG, Lavery LA. Elevated peak plantar pressures in patients who have Charcot arthropathy. J Bone Joint Surg Am 1998;80:365–9.

25. Shem KL. Neuroarthropathy of the wrist in paraplegia: a case report. J Spinal Cord Med 2006;29:436–9.
26. Brown C, Jones B, Akmakijian J, et al. Neuropathic (Charcot) arthropathy of the spine after traumatic spinal paraplegia. Spine 1992;17:S103–8.
27. Smith DG, Barnes BC, Sands AK, et al. Prevalence of radiographic foot abnormalities in patients with diabetes. Foot Ankle Int 1997;18:342–6.
28. Stuck RM, Sohn MW, Budiman-Mak E, et al. Charcot arthropathy risk elevation in the obese diabetic population. Am J Med 2008;121:1008–14.
29. Jones CW, Agolley D, Burns K, et al. Charcot neuroarthropathy presenting with primary bone resorption. Foot 2012;22:258–63.
30. Papanas N, Papatheodorou K, Papazoglou D, et al. Foot temperature in type 2 diabetic patients with or without peripheral neuropathy. Exp Clin Endocrinol Diabetes 2009;117:44–7.
31. Osterhoff G, Böni T, Berli M. Recurrence of acute Charcot neuropathic osteoarthropathy after conservative treatment. Foot Ankle Int 2013;34:359.
32. Petrova NL, Edmonds ME. Charcot neuro-osteoarthropathy—current standards. Diabetes Metab Res Rev 2008;24:S58–61.
33. Chantelau E. The perils of procrastination: effects of early vs. delayed detection and treatment of incipient Charcot fracture. Diabet Med 2005;22:1707–12.
34. Shibata T, Tada K, Hashizume C. The results of arthrodesis of the ankle for leprotic neuroarthropathy. J Bone Joint Surg Am 1990;72A:749–56.
35. Foster AV. Problems with the nomenclature of Charcot's osteoarthropathy. Diabet Foot Ankle 2005;8:37–9.
36. Mabilleau G, Edmonds ME. Role of neuropathy on fracture healing in Charcot neuro-osteoarthropathy. J Musculoskelet Neuronal Interact 2010;10:84–91.
37. Zampa V, Bargellini I, Rizzo L, et al. Role of dynamic MRI in the follow-up of acute Charcot foot in patients with diabetes mellitus. Skeletal Radiol 2011;40:991–9.
38. Ruotolo V, Di Pietro B, Giurato L, et al. A new natural history of Charcot foot: clinical evolution and final outcome of stage 0 Charcot neuroarthropathy in a tertiary referral diabetic foot clinic. Clin Nucl Med 2013;38:506–9.
39. Butalia S, Palda VA, Sargeant RJ, et al. Does this patient with diabetes have osteomyelitis of the lower extremity? JAMA 2008;299:806–13.
40. Tan PL, Teh J. MRI of the diabetic foot: differentiation of infection from neuropathic change. Br J Radiol 2007;80:939–48.
41. Rogers LC, Bevilacqua NJ. Imaging of the Charcot foot. Clin Podiatr Med Surg 2008;25:263–74.
42. Höpfner S, Krolak C, Kessler S, et al. Preoperative imaging of Charcot neuroarthropathy: does the additional application of (18)F-FDG-PET make sense? Nuklearmedizin 2006;45:15–20.
43. Basu S, Chryssikos T, Houseni M, et al. Potential role of FDG PET in the setting of diabetic neuro-osteoarthropathy: can it differentiate uncomplicated Charcot's neuroarthropathy from osteomyelitis and soft-tissue infection? Nucl Med Commun 2007;28:465–72.
44. Ranachowska C, Lass P, Korzon-Burakowska A, et al. Diagnostic imaging of the diabetic foot. Nucl Med Rev Cent East Eur 2010;13:18–22.
45. Zhuang H, Duarte PS, Pourdehand M, et al. Exclusion of chronic osteomyelitis with F-18 fluorodeoxyglucose positron emission tomographic imaging. Clin Nucl Med 2000;25:281–4.
46. Bolouri C, Merwald M, Huellner MW, et al. Performance of orthopantomography, planar scintigraphy, CT alone and SPECT/CT in patients with suspected osteomyelitis of the jaw. Eur J Nucl Med Mol Imaging 2013;40:411–7.

47. Wu JS, Gorbachova T, Morrison WB, et al. Imaging-guided bone biopsy for osteomyelitis: are there factors associated with positive or negative cultures? Am J Roentgenol 2007;188:1529–34.

48. Weiner RD, Viselli SJ, Fulkert KA, et al. Histology versus microbiology for accuracy in identification of osteomyelitis in the diabetic foot. J Foot Ankle Surg 2011; 50:197–200.

49. Pinzur MS, Lio T, Posner M. Treatment of Eichenholtz stage I Charcot foot arthropathy with a weight bearing total contact cast. Foot Ankle Int 2006;27: 324–9.

50. de Souza LJ. Charcot arthropathy and immobilization in a weight-bearing total contact cast. J Bone Joint Surg Am 2008;90A:754–9.

51. Clohisy DR, Thompson RC. Fractures associated with neuropathic arthropathy in adults who have juvenile-onset diabetes. J Bone Joint Surg Am 1988;70: 1192–200.

52. Sinacore DR. Acute Charcot arthropathy in patients with diabetes mellitus: healing times by foot location. J Diabetes Complications 1998;12:287–93.

53. Christensen TM, Gade-Rasmussen B, Pedersen LW. Duration of off-loading and recurrence rate in Charcot osteoarthropathy treated with less restrictive regimen with removable walker. J Diabetes Complications 2012;26:430–4.

54. Bem R, Jirkovská A, Fejfarová V, et al. Intranasal calcitonin in the treatment of acute Charcot neuroosteoarthropathy: a randomized controlled trial. Diabetes Care 2006;29:1392–4.

55. Jude EB, Selby PL, Burgess J, et al. Bisphosphonates in the treatment of Charcot neuroarthropathy: a double-blind randomised controlled trial. Diabetologia 2001;44:2032–7.

56. Pakarinen T, Laine H, Maenpaa H, et al. The effect of zoledronic acid on the clinical resolution of Charcot neuroarthropathy: a pilot randomized controlled trial. Diabetes Care 2011;34:1514–6.

57. Pakarinen TK, Laine HJ, Mäenpää H, et al. Effect of immobilization, off-loading and zoledronic acid on bone mineral density in patients with acute Charcot neuroarthropathy: a prospective randomized trial. Foot Ankle Surg 2013;19:121–4.

58. Richard J, Almasri M, Schuldiner S. Treatment of acute Charcot foot with bisphosphonates: a systematic review of the literature. Diabetologia 2012;55: 1258–64.

59. Bates M, Petrova NL, Edmonds ME. How long does it take to progress from cast to shoes in the management of Charcot osteoarthropathy? Diabet Med 2006;23: 27–A100.

60. Fabrin J, Larsen K, Holstein PE. Long-term follow-up in diabetic Charcot feet with spontaneous onset. Diabetes Care 2000;23:796–800.

61. Sanders L, Frykberg RG. Diabetic neuropathic osteoarthropathy. New York: Livingstone; 1993.

62. Eichenholtz SN. Charcot joints. Springfield (IL): Charles C. Thomas; 1963.

63. Rogers LC, Frykberg RG, Armstrong DG, et al. The Charcot foot in diabetes. J Am Podiatr Med Assoc 2011;101:437–46.

64. Trepman E, Nihal A, Pinzur MS. Current topics review: Charcot neuroarthropathy of the foot and ankle. Foot Ankle Int 2005;26:46–63.

65. Saltzman CL, Hagy ML, Zimmerman B, et al. How effective is intensive nonoperative initial treatment of patients with diabetes and Charcot arthropathy of the feet? Clin Orthop Relat Res 2005;435:185–90.

66. Huang CT, Jackson JR, Moore NB, et al. Amputation: energy cost of ambulation. Arch Phys Med Rehab 1979;60:18–24.

67. Kegel B, Carpenter ML, Burgess EM. Functional capabilities of lower extremity amputees. Arch Phys Med Rehabil 1978;59:109–20.
68. Waters RL, Perry J, Antonelli D, et al. Energy cost of walking amputees: the influence of level of amputation. J Bone Joint Surg Am 1976;58:42–6.
69. Pinzur MS. The metabolic cost of lower extremity amputation. Clin Podiatr Med Surg 1997;14:599–602.
70. Sinacore D, Gutekunst D, Hastings M, et al. Neuropathic midfoot deformity: associations with ankle and subtalar joint motion. J Foot Ankle Res 2013;6:11.
71. Garchar D, DiDomenico L, Klaue K. Reconstruction of Lisfranc joint dislocations secondary to Charcot neuroarthropathy using a plantar plate. J Foot Ankle Surg 2013;52:295–7.
72. Brodsky JW. Management of Charcot joints of the foot and ankle in diabetes. Semin Arthroplasty 1992;3:58–62.
73. Pope E, Takemoto R, Kummer F, et al. Midfoot fusion: a biomechanical comparison of plantar planting vs. intramedullary screws. Foot Ankle Int 2013;34:409.
74. Brodsky JW, Rouse AM. Exostectomy for symptomatic bony prominences in diabetic Charcot feet. Clin Orthop Relat Res 1993;296:21–6.
75. Garapati R, Weinfeld SB. Complex reconstruction of the diabetic foot and ankle. Am J Surg 2004;187:81S–6S.
76. Johnson JE. Operative treatment of neuropathic arthropathy of the foot and ankle. J Bone Joint Surg Am 1998;80:1700–9.
77. Armstrong DG, Stacpoole-Shea S, Nguyen H, et al. Lengthening of the Achilles tendon in diabetic patients who are at high risk for ulceration of the foot. J Bone Joint Surg Am 1999;81:535–8.
78. Lin SS, Lee TH, Wapner KL. Plantar forefoot ulceration with equines deformity of the ankle in diabetic patients: the effect of tendo Achilles lengthening and total contact casting. Orthopedics 1996;19:465–75.
79. Mueller MJ, Sinacore DR, Hastings MK, et al. Effect of Achilles tendon lengthening on neuropathic plantar ulcers. A randomized clinical trial. J Bone Joint Surg Am 2003;85:1436–45.
80. Hollawell SM. Allograft cellular bone matrix as an alternative to autograft in hind foot and ankle fusion procedures. J Foot Ankle Surg 2012;51:222–5.
81. Grant WP, Garcia-Lavin S, Sabo R. Beaming the columns for Charcot diabetic foot reconstruction: a retrospective analysis. J Foot Ankle Surg 2011;50:182–9.
82. Sammarco VJ. Superconstructs in the treatment of Charcot foot deformity: plantar plating, locked plating, and axial screw fixation. Foot Ankle Clin 2009; 14:393–407.
83. Pinzur MS. Neutral ring fixation for high-risk nonplantigrade Charcot midfoot deformity. Foot Ankle Int 2007;28:961–6.
84. Zarutsky E, Rush SM, Schuberth JM. The use of circular wire external fixation in the treatment of salvage ankle arthrodesis. J Foot Ankle Surg 2005;44:22–31.
85. Conway JD. Charcot salvage of the foot and ankle using external fixation. Foot Ankle Clin 2008;13:157–73.
86. Lamm BM, Gottlieb HD, Paley D. A two-stage percutaneous approach to Charcot diabetic foot reconstruction. J Foot Ankle Surg 2010;49:517–22.
87. Altindas M, Kilic A, Ceber M. A new limb-salvaging technique for the treatment of late stage complicated Charcot foot deformity: two-staged Boyd's operation. Foot Ankle Surg 2012;18:190–4.
88. Simon SR, Tejwani SG, Wilson DL, et al. Arthrodesis as an early alternative to nonoperative management of Charcot arthropathy of the diabetic foot. J Bone Joint Surg Am 2000;82:939–50.

89. Wiewiorski M, Yasui T, Miska M, et al. Solid bolt fixation of the medial column in Charcot midfoot arthropathy. J Foot Ankle Surg 2013;52:88–94.

90. Marks RM, Parks BG, Schon LC. Midfoot fusion technique for neuroarthropathic feet: biomechanical analysis and rationale. Foot Ankle Int 1998;19: 507–10.

91. Pinzur MS, Sostak J. Surgical stabilization on nonplantigrade Charcot arthropathy of the midfoot. Am J Orthop 2007;36:361–5.

92. Schon LC, Easley ME, Cohen I, et al. The acquired midtarsus deformity classification system—interobserver reliability and intraobserver reproducibility. Foot Ankle Int 2002;23:30–6.

93. Daver NG, Shelburne SA, Atmar RL, et al. Oral step-down therapy is comparable to intravenous therapy for *Staphylococcus aureus* osteomyelitis. J Infect 2007;54:539–44.

94. Jeffcoate WJ, Lipsky BA. Controversies in diagnosing and managing osteomyelitis of the foot in diabetes. Clin Infect Dis 2004;39:S115–22.

95. Hanssen AD. Local antibiotic delivery vehicles in the treatment of musculoskeletal infection. Clin Orthop Relat Res 2005;437:91–6.

96. Samuel S, Ismavel R, Boopalan PR, et al. Practical considerations in the making and use of high-dose antibiotic-loaded bone cement. Acta Orthop Belg 2010; 76:543–5.

97. Shinsako K, Okui Y, Matsuda Y, et al. Effects of bead size and polymerization in PMMA bone cement on vancomycin release. Biomed Mater Eng 2008;18: 377–85.

98. Ferraris S, Miola M, Bistolfi A, et al. In vitro comparison between commercially and manually mixed antibiotic-loaded bone cements. J Appl Biomater Biomech 2010;8:166–74.

99. Moojen DJ, Hentenaar B, Charles Vogely H, et al. In vitro release of antibiotics from commercial PMMA beads and articulating hip spacers. J Arthroplasty 2008;23:1152–6.

100. Chang Y, Chen WC, Hsieh PH, et al. In vitro activities of daptomycin-, vancomycin-, and teicoplanin-loaded polymethylmethacrylate against methicillin-susceptible, methicillin-resistant, and vancomycin-intermediate strains of *Staphylococcus aureus*. Antimicrob Agents Chemother 2011;55:5480–4.

101. Zgonis T, Stapleton JJ, Roukis TS. A stepwise approach to the surgical management of severe diabetic foot infections. Foot Ankle Spec 2008;1:46–53.

102. Farber DC, Juliano PJ, Cavanagh PR, et al. Single stage correction with external fixation of the ulcerated foot in individuals with Charcot neuroarthropathy. Foot Ankle Int 2002;23:130–4.

103. Saltzman CL. Salvage of diffuse ankle osteomyelitis by single-stage resection and circumferential frame compression arthrodesis. Iowa Orthop J 2005;25: 47–52.

104. Pawar A, Dikmen G, Fragomen A, et al. Antibiotic-coated nail for fusion of infected Charcot Ankles. Foot Ankle Int 2013;34:80–4.

105. Dalla Paola L, Brocco E, Ceccacci T, et al. Limb salvage in Charcot foot and ankle osteomyelitis: combined use single/double stage of arthrodesis and external fixation. Foot Ankle Int 2009;30:1065–70.

106. El-Gafary KA, Mostafa KM, Al-Adly WY. The management of Charcot joint disease affecting the ankle and foot by arthrodesis controlled by an Ilizarov frame: early results. J Bone Joint Surg Br 2009;91:1322–5.

107. Pinzur M, Gil J, Belmares J. Deformity, and maintenance with ring fixation treatment of osteomyelitis in Charcot foot with single-stage resection of infection,

correction of deformity, and maintenance with ring fixation. Foot Ankle Int 2012; 33:1069.

108. Pinzur MS, Gurza E, Kristopaitis T, et al. Hospitalist-orthopedic co-management of high-risk patients undergoing lower extremity reconstruction surgery. Orthopedics 2009;32:495.

109. Wukich DK, Pearson KT. Self-reported outcomes of trans-tibial amputations for non-reconstructable Charcot neuroarthropathy in patients with diabetes: a preliminary report. Diabet Med 2013;30:e87–90.

110. Gil J, Schiff A, Pinzur M. Cost comparison: limb salvage versus amputation in diabetic patients with Charcot foot. Foot Ankle Int 2013;34:1097–9.

Prosthetic Options Available for the Diabetic Lower Limb Amputee

Gautham Chitragari, MBBS[a], David B. Mahler, CPO[b],
Brandon J. Sumpio, BS[c], Peter A. Blume, DPM[b],
Bauer E. Sumpio, MD, PhD[a],*

KEYWORDS

- Lower limb prosthesis • Prosthetic knee • Prosthetic feet
- Recent advances in prosthesis • Power knee • Proprio foot • iWALK

KEY POINTS

- Despite advances in medicine, lower limb amputation still remains as a major complication of diabetes.
- Main components of prosthesis include socket, shank or pylon and the foot.
- Manual locking knee, single axis constant friction knee, polycentric knee, fluid control knee and microprocessor controlled knees are the types of prosthetic knees available.
- Prosthetic feet are classified into solid ankle cushioned heel foot, single axis foot, multi-axis foot and microprocessor foot.
- Partial foot amputation prosthesis include toe fillers, forefoot fillers, ankle orthosis and silicone partial feet.

INTRODUCTION

Although the rate of lower limb amputation in patients with diabetes is decreasing (3.3 per 1000 in 2009 compared with 8.9 per 1000 patients with diabetes in 1990), amputation still remains a major complication of diabetes. The average age-adjusted rates of toe, foot, below-knee, and above-knee amputations between the years 2000 and 2009 were 2.33, 0.7, 1.34, and 0.61 per 1000 diabetic patients, respectively.[1]

Prosthetics have been long used to help amputees ambulate. Arguably, the sacred Indian hymn, "Rig Veda" contains the first written record (between 3500 and 1800 BC) of a lower limb amputation and the use of an iron prosthesis.[2] Most of the

[a] Section of Vascular Surgery, Department of Surgery, Yale University School of Medicine, 333 Cedar Street, New Haven, CT 06510, USA; [b] Orthopedics and Rehabilitation, and Anesthesia, Yale University School of Medicine, 333 Cedar Street, New Haven, CT 06510, USA; [c] Department of surgery, Yale University School of Medicine, 333 Cedar Street, New Haven, CT 06510, USA
* Corresponding author. Yale University School of Medicine, 333 Cedar Street, BB 204, New Haven, CT 06520-8062.
E-mail address: bauer.sumpio@yale.edu

Clin Podiatr Med Surg 31 (2014) 173–185
http://dx.doi.org/10.1016/j.cpm.2013.09.008
0891-8422/14/$ – see front matter © 2014 Elsevier Inc. All rights reserved.
podiatric.theclinics.com

developments in amputation technique and prosthetic design occurred during wars. One of the first recorded design and use of prosthesis in the modern era was in France in 1579 AD by French military surgeon Ambroise Paré.[3] Many improvements in prosthetics over the last decade have occurred with the enhanced understanding of the mechanics of ambulation and improved use of technology. The purpose of this article is to review the different types of prosthetic options available for below knee, ankle, and foot amputees, emphasizing the latest advances in prosthetic design.

The location of amputation and the length of the residuum determine the quality of ambulation with prosthesis.[4–6] As the length of the residual limb decreases, the energy spent to ambulate increases and the velocity of walking decreases. Although the relative energy cost of ambulation (rate of oxygen uptake divided by the individual's maximum ability to perform aerobic exercise) for an above knee amputee is 63%, it is only 42% for a below-knee amputee.[7] Heart rate and oxygen consumption while walking for transtibial amputees is 16% more, even though the velocity of walking is 11% lower than in able-bodied controls.[8] Hence, it is important to attempt to preserve the lowest level of amputation to optimize the quality of ambulation postamputation.

PROSTHESIS

Almost all lower limb prostheses have 3 basic components: a socket, a shank (shin), and a foot (**Fig. 1**).

Socket

The socket is the interface between the prosthesis and the residual limb that serves to deliver the forces associated with various stages of ambulation to the residual limb. The socket should be properly designed to achieve optimal load transmission. Poorly designed sockets not only fail to transmit forces effectively but also produce skin abrasions and much discomfort to the amputee. Ideally, every socket should be custom-made according to the shape, size, and condition of the limb and the degree of mobility required. Currently, custom-made sockets are made using computer-aided design and computer-aided manufacturing, which not only helps in design, but also provides quantitative information regarding load transfer between the socket and the residual limb that helps in objective evaluation of the fit.[9]

Two types of transtibial sockets are available (**Fig. 2**). The patellar tendon-bearing (PTB) socket, developed more than 50 years ago, promotes increased weight-bearing

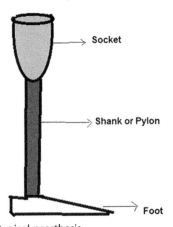

Fig. 1. Different parts of a typical prosthesis.

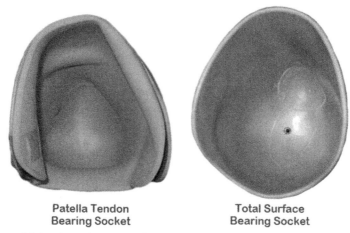

Patella Tendon
Bearing Socket

Total Surface
Bearing Socket

Fig. 2. Transtibial sockets. (*Courtesy of* AustPAR; with permission.)

in the area of the patellar tendon. However, many patients using the PTB socket complain of excessive pressure on the patellar tendon, limited knee flexion, development of skin abrasions, adventitious bursae, and dermatitis.[10,11] Modified versions of PTB sockets like PTB-supracondylar (PTB-SC) and PTB-supracondylar suprapatellar (PTB-SCSP) sockets are available. PTB-SC socket provides improved mediolateral stability by virtue of the high sidewalls. PTB-SCSP, on the other hand, extends further proximally and encloses the patella. PTB-SCSP socket limits the hyperextension of the knee during stance by applying force above the patella, which provides some sensory feedback.

Total surface-bearing (TSB) socket, on the other hand uses suction and distributes weight over the entire stump circumference with less pressure against the patellar tendon. The TSB socket is sensitive to size changes in the stump. Discomfort during knee flexion and excessive sweating in the socket area are a few disadvantages associated with TSB socket.[12]

Liners and Sleeves

Liners and sleeves are additional components in the prosthetic apparatus. A liner is a sock-like, fabricated material used for cushioning the stump and provides volume matching.[13] A suspension sleeve provides friction that improves the adherence of the socket to the stump. Materials like silicone, cell-foam urethanes, and silicone gels are usually used to make liners and sleeves.

Three types of liners are available in the market (**Fig. 3**). They include the cushioning liners, locking liners, and the latest seal-in liners. Cushioning liners are used to provide padding to stumps with scarce soft tissue or bony prominence. Locking liners like the ICEROSS (Icelandic Roll-On Silicone Socket; Ossur, Foothill Ranch, CA, USA) comfort liner (see **Fig. 3**B) contain a pin at the base of the liner that meets with a lock in the socket. ICEROSS Comfort is a prefabricated closed-end liner that has to be turned inside out and then rolled up over the knee. The socket is then pulled over the liner and secured with a shuttle lock using the pin at the end of the liner.

Seal-in liners, like the ICEROSS seal-in X5 (Ossur) (see **Fig. 3**C), are a new type of liners that possess a sealing membrane that conforms to the inside of the socket. These liners produce suction by using a valve mechanism to let the air out. Suspension sleeves use suction or locking mechanism. Sleeves may be made of fabric, gel, or both. Fabric sleeves provide friction between the residuum and the top of the prosthesis. Gel-type

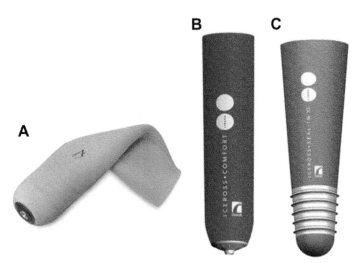

Fig. 3. (*A*) Seal in liner (*Courtesy of* ALPS, St. Petersburg, FL; with permission). (*B*) ICEROSS comfort (*Courtesy of* Ossur Americas, Inc., Foothill Ranch, CA; with permission). (*C*) ICEROSS seal-in X5 transfemoral liner (*Courtesy of* Ossur Americas, Inc., Foothill Ranch, CA; with permission).

sleeves in addition provide an airtight seal. Similar to sockets, prosthetic liners and sleeves provide some discomfort to the amputee with retention of heat and moisture.[14]

Suspension System

To prevent sockets from falling off the residuum, suspension systems are required while using prosthesis. Available methods include self-suspension, suspension devices, and suction suspension. Self-suspension socket conforms to the shape of the residuum and stays intact by itself. Suspension devices use sleeves or belts. Suction suspension uses a suction liner or a suction socket.

Shank

The shank or pylon is a cylindrical tube that connects the socket to the foot. The main function of a shank is to transmit the weight of the amputee to the foot and to the floor. Shanks range from simple static tubes to shells containing motion sensors that provide feedback to the microprocessor in the prosthesis. Some shanks can store and release energy during ambulation.

Shanks are divided into 2 categories based on the part that transfers most of the load. An ectoskeletal or crustacean shank carries forces through its hard outer walls that match the contour of the normal limb. An endoskeletal (modular) shank carries forces through a metallic central skeleton externally covered by a soft covering and is suitable for light to moderate activity. Ectoskeletal shanks provide a natural appearance and are suitable for heavy duty. However, they require careful maintenance.

BELOW-KNEE PROSTHESES

As previously described, each level of amputation requires a different type of prosthesis. Because toe, foot, and below-knee amputations constitute the most amputations performed,[1] this article is limited to the description of prostheses used after those procedures.

Several different types of knee prostheses are available (**Table 1**).

Table 1
The comparison of different prosthetic knees

Model	Advantages	Disadvantages	Indications
Manual locking knee	Inexpensive Higher stability	Awkward gait Does not allow faster cadence Requires manual control	Elderly patients Hemiplegic patients
Single-axis knee, friction-controlled knee	Simple Reliable Low maintenance	Not useful on irregular surfaces Single cadence only	Patients who desire single cadence with restricted access to health care Children
Polycentric knee	Increased stability in stance phase Increased ease of knee flexion during the preswing phase Better cosmetic appearance while sitting Can be used on uneven surfaces	Heavy weight Expensive	Transfemoral amputees with a small stump
Fluid control knee (pneumatic)	Allows changes in speed Stable at any temperature	Less precise than hydraulic knee	Can be used by patients of any age, specially with higher exercise
Fluid control knee (hydraulic)	Allows changes in speed More precise than pneumatic knee	Sensitive to cold temperature Heavier	Can be used by patients of any age, especially with higher exercise demands
Microprocessor knee	Allows higher velocities Energy-saving and provides natural appearing gait Very precise control	Expensive	Patients in excellent physical condition
Power knee	Precise control of walking Propulsion from sitting to standing position	Expensive	Almost anyone

Modified from Tang PC, Ravji K, Key JJ, et al. Let them walk! Current prosthesis options for leg and foot amputees. J Am Coll Surg 2008;206(3):548–60; with permission.

Manual Locking Knee

In this device (**Fig. 4**A), the amputee locks the knee during ambulation and releases the lock to sit, thus enabling a moderate walking speed with comparatively less cardiac effort. The chief disadvantage is the awkward gait that it produces because of the stiff leg. The manual locking knee is best suited for weak amputees desiring a steady gait.

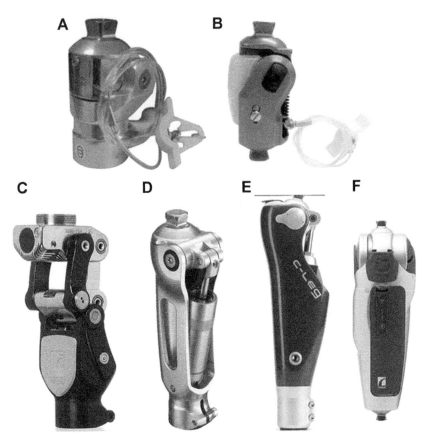

Fig. 4. (A) Manual locking Knee (*Courtesy of* ST&G Corp, Brea, CA; with permission). (B) Single-axis knee (*Courtesy of* ST&G Corp, Brea, CA; with permission). (C) Polycentric knee (*Courtesy of* Ossur Americas, Inc., Foothill Ranch, CA; with permission). (D) Hydraulic knee (*Courtesy of* Ossur Americas, Inc., Foothill Ranch, CA; with permission). (E) C-Leg (*Courtesy of* Ottobock, Plymouth, MN; with permission). (F) Power knee (*Courtesy of* Ossur Americas, Inc., Foothill Ranch, CA; with permission).

Single-Axis, Constant Friction Knee

In this prosthesis (see **Fig. 4**B), flexion and extension occur around a single axis with a friction-based system to provide swing control. Sometimes a spring mechanism is used to promote full leg extension before heel strike. Although it is a simple, reliable, cheap, and low-maintenance device, the friction swing control functions only in one cadence (walking speed). It does not work well on irregular surfaces, owing to poor toe clearance. Except in a few developing countries, this device is rarely used. A modified version of single-axis knee with a braking system is the weight-activated stance control knee or safety knee, whereby the weight of the amputee provides stability during the stance phase and prevents buckling. The amputee is forced to take off his weight to allow the knee to bend while initiating the swing phase or while sitting. Despite the disadvantages such as allowing single cadence and inability to walk on irregular surfaces, this prosthesis is a simple and reliable design. It is best suited for patients with limited access to health care.[15]

Polycentric Axis Knee

Polycentric knee (see **Fig. 4C**), also called as the 4-bar linkage design, consists of 4 points of rotation connected by linkage bars and provides excellent stabilization during stance phase and increased ease of knee flexion during the preswing phase. It also provides better symmetry of walking, a faster walking speed, and natural and better cosmetic appearance while sitting because it causes minimal extrusion of the knee until 90° of flexion.[16] This device allows a mild decrease in prosthetic length and shifts the center of rotation anteriorly when the knee is minimally flexed. This device not only provides increased stability while walking at a moderate pace, but also decreases the risk of stumbling while walking on uneven surfaces. The chief disadvantages of this prosthesis include its heavy weight and increased cost. This device is best suited for short transfemoral amputees and those who desire stance phase stability.

Fluid Control Knees

Fluid control knees contain either air (pneumatic device) or liquid (hydraulic device) to allow variance in walking speed. As the person walks, the air gets progressively compressed and transfers from one piston to the other,[17] providing a nonlinear resistance that controls the speed at which the shin swings forward or backward. Pneumatic devices are best suited for patients who vary their walking speed. However, very high speeds may damage this device.

Unlike pneumatic devices, liquid-based devices (see **Fig. 4D**) allow high ambulation speeds, but are sensitive to cold environments. The system is based on hydraulic dampers that restrict the flow of an incompressible fluid, like silicone oil through a small orifice, which results in change in resistance. Increased cost, weight, and the need for heavy maintenance are some of the disadvantages of the hydraulic knee. Hydraulic knees could be combined with single-axis or multi-axis systems.

Microprocessor Controlled or "Intelligent Knee"

These knees use state-of-the-art technology and allow patients to ambulate at higher cadence with less energy with a precise control of the biomechanics. Microprocessor knees use either hydraulic and/or pneumatic mechanism or magneto-rheological mechanisms to control knee flexion. Unlike the conventional hydraulic knees where the size of the orifice through which the liquid flows changes with friction, the intelligent knee incorporates a microprocessor in the knee joint that detects the swing speed of the patient using sensors and continuously sends signals to the stepper motor. In turn, the stepper motor adjusts the size of the valve in the pneumatic cylinder that finally controls the resistance of the knee. Most of the microprocessor knees calculate the average speed or use the speed of the last few steps to control knee flexion. Examples include the Power knee by Ossur (Ossur; see **Fig. 4F**), Endolite intelligent prosthesis plus by Chas Blatchford & Sons (Basingstoke, United Kingdom), and the highly advanced C-Leg by Otto Bock (Minneapolis, MN, USA) (see **Fig. 4E**). Using the C-leg, the patient can walk downstairs and walk at higher speeds safely. The C-leg uses sensors, which not only detect vertical loading amplitude and saggital knee movement but also the angular acceleration and direction of the knee joint at least 50 times per second which allow it to precisely control the knee's flexion. Several studies have shown enhanced function, ease of performance, and safety of C-leg compared with other types of microprocessor and nonmicroprocessor controlled prosthetic knees.[18,19]

The Rheo leg developed by Ossur is an example of a magneto-rheological knee. These devices use small magnetic particles suspended in a carrier fluid. In the absence of magnetic field, the particles are randomly distributed in the fluid. On application of the magnetic field, these particles align themselves in the direction of the magnetic field that changes the viscosity of the fluid.[20] Rheo leg's microprocessor detects the walking speed as many as 1000 times a second and adjusts the magnetic field using a computerized system. The result is a constant change in the viscosity of the fluid and the joint stiffness according to the walking speed, which allows a smooth gait. Although the microprocessor knees have many advantages, the extremely high cost precludes their use by many amputees.

Power Knee

Power knee by Ossur is the first motor-powered prosthetic knee. In this design, many mechanosensors relay information to a microprocessor. The microprocessor, depending on the phase of the gait cycle and position of the limb, decides the position the knee has to take. It then sends information to the motor, which moves the knee to the desired position. Although research data on the performance of power knee is scant, a recent report showed enhanced symmetry and reduced contralateral hip and knee moments compared with the C-leg.[21] Controlled swing flexion and extension provide increased toe clearance and prevent knee buckling and falls. Power knee also provides powered propulsion to stand from sitting position. The superior accuracy and control enable ambulation in amputees who could not walk even with a microprocessor knee. As with microprocessor knees, the major disadvantage of power knee is the high cost.

PROSTHETIC ANKLE AND FOOT

In the able-bodied person, the foot serves as a shock absorber and provides a stable weight-bearing surface and forward propulsion. The ankle stores energy in the stance phase and returns nearly 540% more energy during push-off.[22] The ideal prosthetic foot is expected to perform similar functions while being light in weight, cheap, and cosmetically acceptable.

Prosthetic feet are classified based on their mobility and their energy-returning ability. The solid ankle cushioned heel (SACH) foot, single-axis foot and multi-axis foot are classified as non-energy-returning and all other designs are classified as energy-returning feet.

Nonenergy Returning Feet

Non-energy-returning feet, as the name suggests, do not release energy during push-off.

SACH

SACH foot (**Fig. 5**A) is a nonarticulating and non-energy-returning prosthetic foot design comprising of a rigid wooden keel enclosed in foam and a compressible heel wedge. Depending on the weight of the amputee and softness of the heel, a pseudo-plantarflexion is produced after heel strike. Although this inexpensive design consumes lot of energy, it is still the most commonly used foot in developing countries.

Single-axis foot

Single-axis foot (see **Fig. 5**B) is an articulating and a non-energy-returning foot that allows movement in one plane. It allows plantar and dorsiflexion around a transverse axis but does not allow any lateral flexion. The degree of plantar flexion and dorsiflexion is controlled by 2 rubber bumpers, which simulate the action of anatomic dorsal and plantar flexors. As the foot plantar flexes, the posteriorly located dorsiflexion bumper is compressed, which resists further plantar flexion. The plantar flexion bumper works in a similar fashion and resists excessive dorsiflexion. The single-axis foot is heavier than the SACH foot, expensive, and requires frequent maintenance of the bumpers.

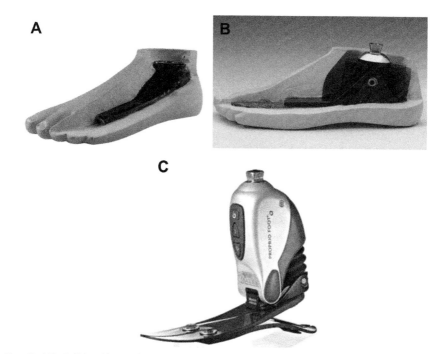

Fig. 5. (A) Solid-ankle cushion heel foot (*Courtesy of* WillowWood, Mt Sterling, OH; with permission). (B) Single-axis foot (*Courtesy of* WillowWood, Mt Sterling, OH; with permission). (C) Proprio foot by Ossur (*Courtesy of* Ossur Americas, Inc., Foothill Ranch, CA; with permission).

Multi-axis foot

Multi-axis foot (see **Fig. 5**C) allows movement in more than one direction. It not only allows plantar flexion and dorsiflexion, but also allows certain degrees of inversion, eversion, and rotation around a vertical axis. Because it allows some rotation, inversion, and eversion, it accommodates to uneven surfaces and absorbs some of the walking stress and thus protects the skin on the residuum while consuming less energy. This foot is best suited for active amputees who require a lot of foot movement. The disadvantages include increased cost, size, weight, and a slight degree of instability in patients with inadequate coordination.

Energy-Returning Feet

Energy-returning feet, also called dynamic response feet, release variable amounts of energy absorbed in stance phase during push-off.[23] A wide range of dynamic response feet are available. Some of them, like the Seattle foot (Model & Instrument Works, Seattle, WA, USA), use a flexible keel covered by polyurethane. The keel gets compressed during mid stance and stores some energy, which is returned during late stance. Examples of energy-returning feet using a similar mechanism include devices like Carbon copy (Ohio Willow Wood, Mt. Sterling, OH, USA) and C-walk (Otto Bock). Although these devices provide some propulsion during push-off by releasing the stored energy, much of the energy is dissipated as heat.

A modified version of the above is the flex foot (Ossur), designed to increase the energy release during push-off. It consists of a carbon fiber shank and a heel spring that allows the compression of both the foot and the shank, unlike the previous device, which allows only foot compression.[24] The advantages include light weight and very low energy consumption. However, high cost prevents many patients from using this.

Microprocessor Feet

Proprio foot

The Proprio foot (Ossur) (**Fig. 5**D) is the first microprocessor prosthetic foot that provides adaptive ankle motion. It has many accelerometers and angle sensors that continuously send information to a microprocessor at a frequency greater than 1000 Hz. The microprocessor optimizes the ankle's angle and position via a linear actuator, depending on the phase of ambulation.[25] The Proprio foot automatically prepositions the foot, dorsiflexes or plantarflexes depending on the terrain, and thus provides superior safety. Adaptive ankle motion minimizes gait deviations because of enhanced foot clearance during swing phase. The energy expenditure of level walking with the Proprio foot was shown to be significantly lower than with dynamic carbon fiber foot.[24] However, no significant difference was found in the energy cost of slope walking by using the adaptive ankle motion of the Proprio foot.[26] The Proprio foot is best suited for patients who desire a natural looking gait, improved symmetry, and balance.

iWALK

iWALK by BiOM, developed at Massachusetts Institute of Technology (Boston, MA, USA) is the first powered prosthetic foot. It has many sensors that detect the trajectory and motion of the prosthesis. The information is sent to a microprocessor, which then sends impulses to a motor to adjust the position and angle of the ankle. Using pattern recognition, the device can detect the approach of a step. Whereas in the Proprio foot, the plantar flexion and dorsiflexion occur only when the foot is unloaded, they occur even when it is loaded in iWALK. Amputees can walk 10% faster and with increased plantar flexion, especially during push-off.[27] Moreover, being a powered foot, iWALK propels the amputee forward during toe-off. All these together drastically decrease the energy expenditure of ambulation. Although data on iWALK are scarce, it is thought that this prosthesis decreases long-term complications, such as socket pain and joint degeneration, as it decreases the stress on other joints.[28]

PARTIAL FOOT AMPUTATION

Partial foot amputation in a patient with diabetes may be performed for peripheral vascular disease–related ischemia or a neuropathy-related nonhealing ulcer of the forefoot. Partial foot amputations are usually performed as salvage procedures to prevent amputation at higher levels. Nevertheless, a significant number of patients end up having a higher level amputation after a partial foot amputation.[29] Partial foot amputations include digital amputation, ray amputation, transmetatarsal amputation, tarsometatarsal amputation (Lisfranc operation), and transtarsal amputations (Chopart amputation).

Toe amputation is the most commonly performed lower limb amputation in patients with diabetes.[1] In a ray amputation, a toe and the corresponding metatarsal bone is amputated as a ray. Deformities caused due to ray or toe amputation depends on the toe or ray amputated. Amputation of the first or fifth toe or ray causes new pressure points and tendon imbalances compared with 2nd, 3rd, and 4th rays. Metatarsal heads are subjected to increased pressure with hallux amputation. However, when compared with a higher level amputation, ray and toe amputations are associated with very few complications and are extremely functional. Most of the prosthetics used for toe amputees consist of a toe filler (**Fig. 6**B). They provide proper shape and prevent shoe deformation. They also provide toe spacing to prevent deviation

A

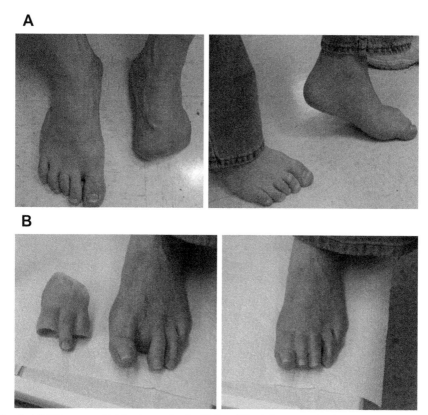

B

Fig. 6. (*A*) Silicone partial foot prosthesis. (*B*) Toe filler (Photo supplied by Alternative Prosthetic Services).

of the other toes toward the center. Ray amputees usually do not require any prosthesis except for first-ray amputation, which is managed by the use of a toe filler.

In metatarsophalyngeal and transmetatarsal amputees, the longitudinal arch of the foot is disrupted. Due to the loss of weight-bearing surface of the foot, the tissues under the metatarsal heads are subjected to excessive pressure, which leads to microtrauma[30]; this is especially important in a diabetic amputee as the patients are usually unaware of the injuries to the foot. Resection of tendon insertions of dorsiflexors during the surgery subjects the foot to unopposed action of triceps surae and gravity,[31] resulting in acquired equinas deformity, which can be prevented either by suturing the tendon ends of dorsiflexors to tarsal bones or by intraoperative Achilles tendon lengthening.[32] Forefoot fillers and inlays are the mainstay of treatment of metatarsophalangeal and transmetatarsal amputees, serving to redistribute the body weight and ground reaction forces on the foot. Most of the time, a carbon graphite plate is placed under the toe filler to reduce the pressure on the residuum.

Midtarsal and tarsometatarsal amputations, in addition to causing increased ground reaction forces and foot pressures, provide a reduced surface area to fit a prosthesis. Usually these amputations require a design that fits proximal to the ankle joint. Most of the times, the ankle-foot orthosis is attached to a forefoot filler. Although these devices lock the ankle, they provide the advantage of redistributing the pressures to a large surface area (the leg). Moreover, they prevent calf atrophy, which is usually seen in partial foot amputees. These prostheses also provide the amputee a sense of push-off at the level of the ankle by using ground reaction forces.

Silicone cosmetic prosthetics are best suited for amputees with fragile skin seeking a better cosmetic outcome. Currently, silicone prostheses (see **Fig. 6**A) are custom-made with matching details of the other foot, like skin color, texture, and hair. Silicone prostheses not only provide excellent cosmesis, but also provide a better functional outcome.[33]

SUMMARY

Lower limb amputation in patients with diabetes is usually a consequence of vascular insufficiency combined with peripheral neuropathy. Although many advances in prosthetic designs were seen in recent years, efficacy of most of them is yet to be completely evaluated. Nevertheless, with improved research in bionics and understanding of the biomechanics of walking, we can foresee the use of near normal prosthetic limb in terms of structure and function in the near future.

REFERENCES

1. Centres for Disease Control and Prevention – Department of Health and Human Services. Crude and Age-Adjusted Hospital Discharge Rates for Nontraumatic Lower Extremity Amputation per 1,000 Diabetic Population, by Level of Amputation (LEA), United States, 1993–2009.
2. Sanders GT. Amputation prosthetics. Philadelphia: FA Davis Company; 1986.
3. Hernigou P. Ambroise pare IV: the early history of artificial limbs (from robotic to prostheses). Int Orthop 2013;37(6):1195–7.
4. Arwert HJ, van Doorn-Loogman MH, Koning J, et al. Residual-limb quality and functional mobility 1 year after transtibial amputation caused by vascular insufficiency. J Rehabil R D 2007;44(5):717–22.
5. Bell JC, Wolf EJ, Schnall BL, et al. Transfemoral amputations: the effect of residual limb length and orientation on gait analysis outcome measures. J Bone Joint Surg Am 2013;95(5):408–14.
6. Tang PC, Ravji K, Key JJ, et al. Let them walk! Current prosthesis options for leg and foot amputees. J Am Coll Surg 2008;206(3):548–60.
7. Waters RL, Perry J, Antonelli D, et al. Energy cost of walking of amputees: the influence of level of amputation. J Bone Joint Surg Am 1976;58(1):42–6.
8. Gailey RS, Wenger MA, Raya M, et al. Energy expenditure of trans-tibial amputees during ambulation at self-selected pace. Prosthet Orthot Int 1994;18(2):84–92.
9. Mak AF, Zhang M, Boone DA. State-of-the-art research in lower-limb prosthetic biomechanics-socket interface: a review. J Rehabil R D 2001;38(2):161–74.
10. Ahmed A, Bayol MG, Ha SB. Adventitious bursae in below knee amputees: case reports and a review of the literature. Am J Phys Med Rehabil 1994;73:124–9.
11. Moo EK, Osman NA, Pingguan-Murphy B, et al. Interface pressure profile analysis for patellar tendon-bearing socket and hydrostatic socket. Acta Bioeng Biomech 2009;11(4):37–43.
12. Hachisuka K, Dozono K, Ogata H, et al. Total surface bearing below-knee prosthesis: advantages, disadvantages, and clinical implications. Arch Phys Med Rehabil 1998;79(7):783–9.
13. Hatfield AG, Morrison JD. Polyurethane gel liner usage in the oxford prosthetic service. Prosthet Orthot Int 2001;25(1):41–6.

14. Hachisuka K, Nakamura T, Ohmine S, et al. Hygiene problems of residual limb and silicone liners in transtibial amputees wearing the total surface bearing socket. Arch Phys Med Rehabil 2001;82(9):1286–90.
15. Michael JW. Modern prosthetic knee mechanisms. Clin Orthop Relat Res 1999;(361):39–47.
16. Taheri A, Karimi MT. Evaluation of the gait performance of above-knee amputees while walking with 3R20 and 3R15 knee joints. J Res Med Sci 2012;17(3):258–63.
17. Buckley JG, Spence WD, Solomonidis SE. Energy cost of walking: comparison of "intelligent prosthesis" with conventional mechanism. Arch Phys Med Rehabil 1997;78:330–3.
18. Bellmann M, Schmalz T, Blumentritt S. Comparative biomechanical analysis of current microprocessor-controlled prosthetic knee joints. Arch Phys Med Rehabil 2010;91(4):644–52.
19. Seymour R, Engbretson B, Kott K, et al. Comparison between the C-leg microprocessor-controlled prosthetic knee and non-microprocessor control prosthetic knees: a preliminary study of energy expenditure, obstacle course performance, and quality of life survey. Prosthet Orthot Int 2007;31(1):51–61.
20. Johansson JL, Sherrill DM, Riley PO, et al. A clinical comparison of variable-damping and mechanically passive prosthetic knee devices. Am J Phys Med Rehabil 2005;84(8):563–75.
21. Highsmith MJ, Kahle JT, Carey SL, et al. Kinetic differences using a power knee and C-leg while sitting down and standing up: a case report. J Pediatr Ophthalmol 2010;22(4):237–43.
22. Winter DA. Energy generation and absorption at the ankle and knee during fast, natural and slow cadences. Clin Orthop Relat Res 1983;175:147–54.
23. Wing DC, Hittenberger DA. Energy-storing prosthetic feet. Arch Phys Med Rehabil 1989;70(4):330–5.
24. Schneider K, Hart T, Zernicke RF, et al. Dynamics of below-knee child amputee gait: SACH foot versus Flex foot. J Biomech 1993;26(10):1191–204.
25. Delussu AS, Brunelli S, Paradisi F, et al. Assessment of the effects of carbon fiber and bionic foot during overground and treadmill walking in transtibial amputees. Gait Posture 2013;38(4):876–82.
26. Darter BJ, Wilken JM. Energetic consequences of using a prosthesis with adaptive ankle motion during slope walking in person with transtibial amputation. Prosthet Orthot Int 2013. [Epub ahead of print March 22nd, 2013].
27. Gates DH, Aldridge JM, Wilken JM. Kinematic comparison of walking on uneven ground using powered and unpowered prostheses. Clin Biomech 2013;28(4):467–72.
28. Mancinelli C, Patritti BL, Tropea P, et al. Comparing a passive-elastic and a powered prosthesis in transtibial amputees. Conf Proc IEEE Eng Med Biol Soc 2011; 2011:8255–8.
29. Armstrong DG, Lavery LA, Harkless LB, et al. Amputation and reamputation of the diabetic foot. J Am Podiatr Med Assoc 1997;87(6):255–9.
30. Mueller MJ, Sinacore DR. Rehabilitation factors following transmetatarsal amputation. Phys Ther 1994;74(11):1027–33.
31. Sanders LJ. Transmetatarsal and midfoot amputations. Clin Podiatr Med Surg 1997;14(4):741–62.
32. Fergason J, Keeling JJ, Bluman EM. Recent advances in lower extremity amputations and prosthetics for the combat injured patient. Foot Ankle Clin 2010;15(1): 151–74.
33. Burger H, Erzar D, Maver T, et al. Biomechanics of walking with silicone prosthesis after midtarsal (Chopart) disarticulation. Clin Biomech 2009;24(6):510–6.

Index

Note: Page numbers of article titles are in **boldface** type.

A

ACCORD (Action to Control Cardiovascular Risk in Diabetes), 20
Action in Diabetes and Vascular Disease (ADVANCE), 20
Action to Control Cardiovascular Risk in Diabetes (ACCORD), 20
ADVANCE (Action in Diabetes and Vascular Disease), 20
Advancement flaps, 131–133
Amputations. *See also* Partial foot amputations.
    prostheses for, **173–185**
Angiosomes, in revascularization, 22
Ankle-brachial index, in peripheral vascular disease, 15–16
Ankle-foot orthosis, 83–85
Antibiotics
    for Charcot neuroarthropathy, 162–163
    for infections, 60, 64–65
Antiplatelet therapy, for peripheral vascular disease, 21
Apligraf BAT, 97–98
Aspirin, for peripheral vascular disease, 21
Atherectomy, for peripheral vascular disease, 23
Autonomic neuropathy, in Charcot neuroarthropathy, 152–154

B

BATs. *See* Bioengineered alternative tissues.
Beta blockers, perioperative, 3, 7
Bilayer bioengineered alternative tissues, 92, 95–98
Bilobed flaps, 137
Bioengineered alternative tissues, **89–101**
    acellular, 92, 95
    cellular, 92
    future of, 98–99
    indications for, 90
    principles of, 90–91
    risks of, 93
    types of, 89–90
Biopsy
    for Charcot neuroarthropathy, 156
    for infections, 60, 62
Bisphosphonates, for Charcot neuroarthropathy, 157
Bone grafts, for Charcot neuroarthropathy, 161
Braces. *See* Offloading options.

Clin Podiatr Med Surg 31 (2014) 187–195
http://dx.doi.org/10.1016/S0891-8422(13)00124-9
0891-8422/14/$ – see front matter © 2014 Elsevier Inc. All rights reserved.

podiatric.theclinics.com

C

Callus, offloading options for, 73
CAPRIE (Clopidogel versus Aspirin in Patients at Risk of Ischemic Events) study, 21
Carbon copy foot, 181
Cardiac disease, perioperative management of, 2–3, 5, 20–21
CARDS (Collaborative Atorvastatin Diabetes Study), 20–21
Cast, total contact, 75, 83, 85, 156–157
Cement, antibiotic-impregnated, for infections, 64–65
Central ray or toe, amputation of, 112–115
Charcot neuroarthropathy, **151–172**
    classification of, 154–155
    complexity of, 164–165
    definition of, 152
    deformity correction algorithm for, 163–164
    diagnosis of, 154–156, 162–163
    etiology of, 152–154
    history of, 151–152
    orthotic walker for, 83
    prevalence of, 152
    recurrence of, 157
    treatment of, 156–164
Chopart amputation, 121–125
Chronic ischemic diabetic foot, **27–42**
    cell therapies for, 28–34
    drugs for, 35–37
    incidence of, 28
    pathophysiology of, 28
    rheologic treatment for, 37–38
Clopidogel versus Aspirin in Patients at Risk of Ischemic Events (CAPRIE) study, 21
Collaborative Atorvastatin Diabetes Study (CARDS), 20–21
Computed tomography, 51–52, 155–156
Computed tomography angiography, for peripheral vascular disease, 17–19
Contraction, of skin grafts, 139–140
C-reactive protein
    in infections, 59
    in peripheral vascular disease, 13
Culture
    for Charcot neuroarthropathy, 156
    for infections, 59, 62
Cultured epithelial autografts (epidermal bioengineered alternative tissues), 92–94
Cushioning liners, of prosthesis, 175–176
C-Walk foot, 181
Cytokines, in Charcot neuroarthropathy, 153–154

D

De Marco formula, for ischemic foot, 37
Debridement
    for infections, 60, 62–63
    of skin graft recipient bed, 140

Dermagraft, 94–96
Dermal bioengineered alternative tissues, 92, 94–96
Dermatome, for skin graft harvesting, 141
Diabetic foot and ankle
    amputations for, **103–126**
    bioengineered tissues for, **89–101**
    Charcot neuropathy of, 83, **151–172**
    chronic ischemia in, **27–42**
    infections of. *See* Infections and osteomyelitis.
    offloading of, **71–88**
    pathology of, 12–13
    perioperative management of, **1–10**
    peripheral vascular disease and, **11–26**
    prosthetic options for, **173–185**
    soft tissue coverage for, **127–150**
Digital subtraction angiography, for peripheral vascular disease, 19
Doppler evaluation, for peripheral vascular disease, 14–18
Double V-to-Y flaps, 132–133
Dressing, for skin graft, 142

E

Ectoskeletal shank, of prosthesis, 176
Eichenholtz stage, of Charcot neuroarthropathy, 157
Electrocardiography, perioperative, 3
Endoskeletal shank, of prosthesis, 176
Endovascular techniques, for peripheral vascular disease, 22–23
Energy-returning feet, 181–182
Epidermal bioengineered alternative tissues, 92–94
Epidex, 94
Erythrocyte sedimentation rate, in infections, 59
Exostectomy, for Charcot neuroarthropathy, 160
External fixation, for Charcot neuroarthropathy, 161–162

F

Femoropopliteal bypass, 21–22
Fifth ray, amputation of, 116–119
First ray, amputation of, 107–112
Fixation, for Charcot neuroarthropathy, 161–162
Flaps, 130–137
    anatomy of, 129
    complications of, 143–144
    decision ladder for, 127
    for amputation coverage, 104–107
    patient health parameters and, 128–129
    physiology of, 130
    principles of, 128
    technique for, 130–131
    types of, 131–137
Flex foot, 181–182

Fluid control knees, 177, 179
Friction-controlled knee, 177

G

Glucose control, perioperative, 6–9, 20
GraftJacket, 95–96
Granulocyte colony-stimulating factor, for ischemic foot, 36

H

Hallux, amputation of, 107–110
Healing, of skin grafts, 138–139, 143–144
Heart Outcomes Prevention Evaluation (HOPE), 20
Heberprot-P, for ischemic foot, 36–37
HELP (heparin-induced extracorporeal low-density lipoprotein precipitation), for ischemic
    foot, 38
Hematoma, in skin graft, 143
Heparin-induced extracorporeal low-density lipoprotein precipitation (HELP), for ischemic
    foot, 38
HOPE (Heart Outcomes Prevention Evaluation), 20
Human epidermal growth factor, for ischemic foot, 36–37
Hydraulic (fluid control) knee, 177, 179
Hypertension, treatment of, 20

I

ICECROSS liners, of prosthesis, 175–176
Imaging, **43–56**. *See also specific modalities.*
    computed tomography, 51–52
    magnetic resonance imaging, 47–51
    radiography, 44, 50
    radionuclide bone scans, 45–47
    single-photon emission computed tomography, 52–53
    ultrasonography, 44
Infections and osteomyelitis, **57–70**
    anatomic considerations in, 61
    diagnosis of, 58–60
    in Charcot neuroarthropathy, 155–156, 162–163
    in peripheral vascular disease, 15
    in skin grafts, 143
    nonoperative treatment of, 60–61
    outcomes of, 65
    pathology of, 58
    prevalence of, 57
    recurrence of, 66
    statistics on, 58
    surgical treatment of, 58–65
    wound closure for, 62–63
Inflammation, uncontrolled, in Charcot neuroarthropathy, 153–154
Infrapopliteal percutaneous transluminal angioplasty, for peripheral vascular disease, 22–23
Insulin, perioperative, 6–9

Insulin resistance, 12–13
Integra, 95–97
Intelligent (microprocessor) knee, 177, 179–180
Intramedullary screws, for Charcot neuroarthropathy, 162
Ischemic diabetic foot. *See* Chronic ischemic diabetic foot.
iWALK prosthetic foot, 182

K

Kidney disease, perioperative management with, 3–5, 7

L

Limberg flaps, 134–135
Liners, of prosthesis, 175–176
Lipoaspirate cell therapy, for ischemic foot, 33–34
Lipo-prostaglandin, for ischemic foot, 35–36
Lisfranc disarticulation, 123
Locking liners, of prosthesis, 175–176

M

Magnetic resonance imaging, 47–51
    for Charcot neuroarthropathy, 155–156
    for infections, 58–59
Magnetic resonance imaging angiography, for peripheral vascular disease, 19
Manual locking knee, 177
Matristem, 96
Meshing, of skin graft, 141–142
Metatarsophalangeal amputation, 183
Microprocessor foot, 182
Microprocessor knee, 177, 179–180
Midfoot amputation, 121–125
Midtarsal amputation, 121–125
Multi-axis foot, 181
Muscle flaps, for infections, 63–64
Myocardial infarction, perioperative, 3, 5
Myskin, 94

N

Negative Pressure Wound Therapy, for skin graft, 142
Nephropathy, perioperative management with, 3–5, 7
Neuropathy, Charcot. *See* Charcot neuroarthropathy.
Neurotraumatic theory, of Charcot neuroarthropathy, 152–153
Neurovascular theory, of Charcot neuroarthropathy, 152–153
Nitric oxide, in peripheral vascular disease, 13
Nonenergy-returning feet, 180–181

O

Oasis BAT, 96
Offloading options, **71–88**
    accommodative, 72
    clinical correlation and, 78–85
    complications of, 85–87
    foot presentations and, 72–78
    for ideal foot, 72–73
    functional, 72
Oral hypoglycemic agents, perioperative, 6
Orcel BAT, 97
Organization phase, of skin graft healing, 139
Orthotics. *See* Offloading options.
Osteomyelitis. *See* Infections and osteomyelitis.

P

Partial foot amputations, **103–126**
    central ray, 112–115
    fifth ray, 116–119
    first ray, 107–112
    hallux, 107–110
    midfoot, 121–125
    options for, 103–104
    procedure for, 104–107
    protheses for, 182–184
    rearfoot, 121–125
    transmetatarsal, 119–121
Patellar tendon-bearing sockets and modifications, of prosthesis, 174–175
Pedal bypass grafts, 21–22
Pedorthic strategies. *See* Offloading options.
Perfusion tests, in peripheral vascular disease, 16
Perioperative management. *See also specific procedures.*
    assessment in, 2
    glucose control in, 6–9, 20
    history in, 4
    in cardiac disease, 2–3
    in kidney disease, 3–5, 7
Peripheral vascular disease, **11–26**
    atypical presentations of, 14
    epidemiology of, 12
    imaging for, 15–19
    pathology of, 12–13
    patient history of, 13–14
    physical examination for, 14–15
    surgical options with, 21–23
    treatment of, 20–23
PermaDerm, 98
Pie-crusting, of skin graft, 141–142
Plantar plating, for Charcot neuroarthropathy, 161–162
Plastizote, for orthotics, 78–80

Plate fixation, for Charcot neuroarthropathy, 161–162
Pneumatic (fluid control) knee, 177, 179
Polycentric axis knee, 177, 179
Polyvinylpyrrolidone, in De Marco formula, 37
Porcine xenograft, 140
Positron emission tomography, for Charcot neuroarthropathy, 155–156
Postoperative periods, offloading options for, 76–78
Power knee, 177, 180
Preoperative period, offloading options for, 76–78
PriMatrix, 95–96
Probe-to-bone test, 15, 59
Procaine, in De Marco formula, 37
Processed lipoaspirate cell therapy, for ischemic foot, 33–34
Proprio foot, 182
Prostaglandins, for ischemic foot, 35–36
Prostheses, **173–185**
    ankle-foot, 180–182
    below-knee, 176–180
    components of, 174–176
    history of, 173–174
    partial-foot, 182–184
Pulse, in peripheral vascular disease, 14–15
Pulse volume recordings, in peripheral vascular disease, 16

R

Radiography, 44, 50, 58–59
Radionuclide bone scans, 45–47, 59
RANKL, in Charcot neuroarthropathy, 153–154
Rearfoot amputation, 121–125
Recanalization, for peripheral vascular disease, 23
Revascularization
    for peripheral vascular disease, 21–23
    for skin graft healing, 138
Rheological treatment, for ischemic foot, 37
Rhomboid flaps, 134–135
Rocker bottom shoes, 80–81
Rotation flaps, 133–134

S

SACH foot, 180
Seal-in liners, of prosthesis, 175–176
Seattle foot, 181
Serum imbibition, in skin graft healing, 138
Shanks, of prosthesis, 176
Shoes
    for partial amputations, 182–184
    therapeutic, 80
Silver sulfasdiazine, for skin graft recipient bed, 140
Single lobe flaps, 136–137

Single rotation flaps, 133–134
Single-axis foot, 180
Single-axis knee, 177–178
Single-photon emission computed tomography, 52–53, 60
Skin grafts, 137–144
    anatomy of, 129
    application of, 142
    complications of, 143–144
    contraction in, 139–140
    decision ladder for, 127
    donor site harvesting of, 141
    dressing for, 142
    for infections, 62–63
    healing of, 138–139, 143–144
    indications for, 140
    meshing, 141–142
    patient health parameters and, 128–129
    physiology of, 138–139
    pie-crusting of, 141–142
    postoperative care for, 142–143
    principles of, 128
    recipient bed preparation for, 140–141
    thickness classification of, 137–138
Sleeves, of prosthesis, 175–176
Socket, of prosthesis, 174–175
Soft tissue coverage, **127–150**. *See also* Flaps; Skin grafts.
    anatomy of, 129
    bioengineered alternative tissues, **89–101**
    decision ladder for, 127
    patient health parameters and, 128–129
    principles of, 128
Stem cell transplantation
    autologous, for ischemic foot, 28–33
    for BAT, 98–99
Stents, for peripheral vascular disease, 23
Stroke, perioperative, 3, 5
Subintimal recanalization, for peripheral vascular disease, 23
Suspension system, of prosthesis, 176
Syme amputation
    distal central ray, 112
    distal hallux, 107–108

T

Tarsometatarsal joint amputation, 123, 183–184
Theraskin, 97–98
Tissuetech, 97–98
Toe amputation, protheses for, 182–184
Total contact cast, 75, 83, 85, 156–157
Total surface-bearing socket, of prosthesis, 175
Transmetatarsal amputation, 119–121, 183–184

Transposition flaps, 134–137
Transtarsal amputation, 121–125
Transtibial sockets, of prosthesis, 174–175

U

UKPDS (United Kingdom Prospective Diabetes Study), 20
Ulcer(s)
    examination of, in peripheral vascular disease, 14–15
    from orthosis, 87
    infected. See Infections and osteomyelitis.
    offloading options for, 73–75
Ultrasonography, 44
    for infections, 58–59
    for peripheral vascular disease, 16–18
United Kingdom Prospective Diabetes Study (UKPDS), 20
Urokinase, for ischemic foot, 37–38

V

VADT (Veterans Affairs Diabetes Trial), 20
Vascular examination, in peripheral vascular disease, 14–15
Vascular failure, in skin graft, 143
Veterans Affairs Diabetes Trial (VADT), 20
V-to-Y flaps, 132

W

Wound closure, bioengineered alternative tissues for, **89–101**

Moving?

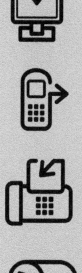

Make sure your subscription moves with you!

To notify us of your new address, find your **Clinics Account Number** (located on your mailing label above your name), and contact customer service at:

Email: journalscustomerservice-usa@elsevier.com

800-654-2452 (subscribers in the U.S. & Canada)
314-447-8871 (subscribers outside of the U.S. & Canada)

Fax number: 314-447-8029

Elsevier Health Sciences Division
Subscription Customer Service
3251 Riverport Lane
Maryland Heights, MO 63043

*To ensure uninterrupted delivery of your subscription, please notify us at least 4 weeks in advance of move.

Printed and bound by CPI Group (UK) Ltd, Croydon, CR0 4YY

03/10/2024

01040409-0001